The Washington Manual™ Geriatrics Subspecialty Consult

W9-BQL-284

The Washington Manual™ Geriatrics Subspecialty Consult

Faculty Advisor
Stanley J. Birge
Associate Professor of Medicine
Department of Internal Medicine
Division of Geriatrics and Nutritional
Science
Washington University School of
Medicine
St. Louis, Missouri

The Washington Manual™ Geriatrics Subspecialty Consult

Editor
Kyle C. Moylan, M.D.
Fellow, Division of Geriatrics and
Nutritional Science
Department of Internal Medicine
Washington University School of Medicine
St. Louis, Missouri

Series Editor
Tammy L. Lin, M.D.
Adjunct Assistant Professor of Medicine
Washington University School of Medicine
St. Louis, Missouri

Series Advisor
Daniel M. Goodenberger, M.D.
Professor of Medicine
Washington University School of Medicine
Chief, Division of Medical Education
Director, Internal Medicine Residency
Program
Barnes-Jewish Hospital
St. Louis, Missouri

LIPPINCOTT WILLIAMS & WILKINS
A **Wolters Kluwer** Company
Philadelphia · Baltimore · New York · London
Buenos Aires · Hong Kong · Sydney · Tokyo

Acquisitions Editors: Danette Somers and James Ryan
Developmental Editors: Scott Marinaro and Keith Donnellan
Supervising Editor: Mary Ann McLaughlin
Production Editor: Brooke Begin, Silverchair Science + Communications
Manufacturing Manager: Colin Warnock
Cover Designer: QT Design
Compositor: Silverchair Science + Communications
Printer: RR Donnelley

Library of Congress Cataloging-in-Publication Data

The Washington manual geriatrics subspecialty consult / editor, Kyle Moylan.
    p. ; cm. -- (The Washington manual subspecialty consult series)
  Includes bibliographical references and index.
  ISBN 0-7817-4379-6
  1. Geriatrics--Handbooks, manuals, etc. I. Moylan, Kyle. II. Series.
  [DNLM: 1. Geriatrics--Handbooks. WT 39 W319 2003]
  RC952.55.W376 2003
  618.97--dc21

                                                    2003044242

The Washington Manual™ is an intent-to-use mark belonging to Washington University in St. Louis to which international legal protection applies. The mark is used in this publication by LWW under license from Washington University.

Care has been taken to confirm the accuracy of the information presented and to describe generally accepted practices. However, the authors, editors, and publisher are not responsible for errors or omissions or for any consequences from application of the information in this book and make no warranty, expressed or implied, with respect to the currency, completeness, or accuracy of the contents of the publication. Application of this information in a particular situation remains the professional responsibility of the practitioner.

The authors, editors, and publisher have exerted every effort to ensure that drug selection and dosage set forth in this text are in accordance with current recommendations and practice at the time of publication. However, in view of ongoing research, changes in government regulations, and the constant flow of information relating to drug therapy and drug reactions, the reader is urged to check the package insert for each drug for any change in indications and dosage and for added warnings and precautions. This is particularly important when the recommended agent is a new or infrequently employed drug.

Some drugs and medical devices presented in this publication have Food and Drug Administration (FDA) clearance for limited use in restricted research settings. It is the responsibility of health care providers to ascertain the FDA status of each drug or device planned for use in their clinical practice.

10 9 8 7 6 5 4 3 2

Contents

Tammy L. Lin

Contributing Authors

Sam B. Bhayani, M.D.

Instructor of Urology
Brady Urological Institute
Johns Hopkins Hospital
Baltimore, Maryland

Stanley J. Birge, M.D.

Associate Professor of Medicine
Department of Internal Medicine
Division of Geriatics and Nutritional
Science
Washington University School of
Medicine
St. Louis, Missouri

David B. Carr, M.D.

Associate Professor of Medicine
Department of Internal Medicine
Division of Geriatrics and Nutritional
Science
Washington University School of
Medicine
St. Louis, Missouri

Susan M. Culican, M.D., Ph.D.

Instructor in Ophthalmology
Washington University School of
Medicine
St. Louis, Missouri

Kellie L. Flood, M.D.

Instructor of Medicine
Department of Internal Medicine
Division of Geriatrics and Nutritional
Science
Washington University School of
Medicine
St. Louis, Missouri

Roger Kerzner, M.D.

Fellow in Cardiology
Department of Internal Medicine
Washington University School of
Medicine
St. Louis, Missouri

Steve R. Lai, M.D.

Geriatric Fellow
Stanford University School of Medicine
Stanford, California
Veterans Affairs Palo Alto
Palo Alto, California

Tammy L. Lin, M.D.

Adjunct Assistant Professor of Medicine
Washington University School of
Medicine
St. Louis, Missouri

Kyle C. Moylan, M.D.

Fellow, Division of Geriatrics and
Nutritional Science
Department of Internal Medicine
Washington University School of
Medicine
St. Louis, Missouri

Rebecca M. Shepherd, M.D.

Fellow, Department of Rheumatology
Washington University School of
Medicine
St. Louis, Missouri

Divya Shroff, M.D.

Resident Physician
Department of Internal Medicine
Washington University School of
Medicine
St. Louis, Missouri

Latha Sivaprasad, M.D.

Instructor of Medicine
Department of Internal Medicine
Division of Cardiology
Washington University School of
Medicine
St. Louis, Missouri

Ulker Tok, M.D.

Fellow, Division of Rheumatology
Department of Internal Medicine
Washington University School of
Medicine
St. Louis, Missouri

Monique Williams, M.D.

Fellow, Division of Geriatrics and
Nutritional Science
Department of Internal Medicine
Washington University School of
Medicine
St. Louis, Missouri

Randall Wooley, M.D.

Physician
Department of Internal Medicine
Presbyterian Hospital of Dallas
Dallas, Texas

Chairman's Note

Medical knowledge is increasing at an exponential rate, and physicians are being bombarded with new facts at a pace that many find overwhelming. The Washington Manual™ Subspecialty Consult Series was developed in this context for interns, residents, medical students, and other practitioners in need of readily accessible practical clinical information. They therefore meet an important unmet need in an era of information overload.

I would like to acknowledge the authors who have contributed to these books. In particular, Tammy L. Lin, M.D., Series Editor, provided energetic and inspired leadership, and Daniel M. Goodenberger,

M.D., Series Advisor, Chief of the Division of Medical Education in the Department of Medicine at Washington University, is a continual source of sage advice. The efforts and outstanding skill of the lead authors are evident in the quality of the final product. I am confident that this series will meet its desired goal of providing practical knowledge that can be directly applied to improving patient care.

Kenneth S. Polonsky, M.D.
Adolphus Busch Professor
Chairman, Department of Medicine
Washington University School of Medicine
St. Louis, Missouri

Series Preface

The Washington Manual™ Subspecialty Consult Series is designed to provide quick access to the essential information needed to evaluate a patient on a subspecialty consult service. Each manual includes the most updated and useful information on commonly encountered symptoms or diseases and highlights the practical information you need to gather before formulating a plan. Special efforts have been made to organize the information so that these guides will be valuable and trusted companions for medical students, residents, and fellows. They cover everything from questions to ask during the initial consult to issues in subsequent management.

One of the strengths of this series is that it is written by residents and fellows who know how busy a consult service can be, who know what information will be most helpful, and who can detail a practical approach to patient care. Each volume is written to provide enough information for you to evaluate a patient until more in-depth reading can be done on a particular topic. Throughout the series, key references are noted, difficult management situations are addressed, and appropriate practice guidelines are included. Another strength of this series is that it was written in concert. All of the guides were designed to work together.

The most important strength of this series is the collection of authors, faculty advisors, and, especially, lead authors assembled to write this series. In addition, we received incredible commitment and support from our chairman, Kenneth S. Polonsky, M.D. As a result, the extraordinary depth of talent and genuine interest in teaching others at Washington University is showcased in this series. Although there has always been house staff involvement in editing The Washington Manual™ series, it came to our attention that many of them also wanted to be involved in writing and making decisions about what to convey to fellow colleagues. Remarkably, many of the lead authors became junior subspecialty fellows while writing their guides. Their desire to pass on what they were learning, while trying to balance multiple responsibilities, is a testament to their dedication and skills as clinicians, teachers, and leaders.

We hope this series fulfills the need for essential and practical knowledge for those learning the art of consultation in a particular subspecialty and for those just passing through it.

Tammy L. Lin, M.D., Series Editor
Daniel M. Goodenberger, M.D.,
Series Advisor

Preface

Welcome to the first edition of The Washington Manual™ Geriatrics Subspecialty Consult. This handbook on geriatrics is intended to serve as a useful resource for medical students, residents, and fellows. Although it is in no way intended to be a comprehensive textbook of geriatric medicine, it does provide a framework for approaching many of the important issues that arise in geriatrics. We have tried to provide the most clinically relevant information, focusing on key aspects of the evaluation and treatment of common geriatric disorders and consultations. When possible, tables and appendixes have been provided for rapid access in the clinical setting.

This publication would not be possible without help from many people. The residents and fellows at Washington University School of Medicine from the fields of internal medicine (Randall Wooley, Divya Shroff, Latha Sivaprasad), geriatrics (Monique Williams, Steve R. Lai—now at Stanford), cardiology (Roger Kerzner with the help of Michael Rich), ophthalmology (Susan M. Culican), rheu-

matology (Rebecca M. Shepherd and Ulker Tok), and urology (Sam B. Bhayani) formed the core driving force behind this publication. Completion of the project would have been impossible without the assistance of faculty from the Division of Geriatrics and Nutritional Science, particularly David B. Carr and Kellie L. Flood. Extra thanks needs to be given to Stanley J. Birge for his invaluable insight, experience, and endless hours reading manuscripts. I would not have been able to undertake this project without the endless support and understanding from my wife, Lesli.

We all hope that practitioners in all fields of medicine find this first edition to be a helpful resource as the health care system prepares for an unprecedented number of older adults. Work on the next edition has already begun to provide up-to-date information and expand the topics covered. Input from readers for future directions of the text is appreciated.

K.C.M.

Key to Abbreviations

AARP	American Association of Retired Persons
ACE	angiotensin-converting enzyme
ASA	aspirin
ATP	adenosine triphosphate
BMI	body mass index
BP	blood pressure
BUN	blood urea nitrogen
CBC	complete blood count
CNS	central nervous system
COPD	chronic obstructive pulmonary disease
Cr	creatinine
CT	computed tomography
DBP	diastolic blood pressure
DSM-IV	*Diagnostic and Statistical Manual of Mental Disorders*, 4th edition
ECG	electrocardiography
EEG	electroencephalography
ER	emergency room
ESR	erythrocyte sedimentation rate
FDA	U.S. Food and Drug Administration
fMRI	functional magnetic resonance imaging
GI	gastrointestinal
Hct	hematocrit
HIV	human immunodeficiency virus
HMG CoA	3-hydroxy-3-methylglutaryl coenzyme A
HTN	hypertension
INR	international normalized ratio
IV	intravenous
MAO	monoamine oxidase
MMSE	Mini-Mental State Examination
MRI	magnetic resonance imaging
NG	nasogastric
NSAIDs	nonsteroidal antiinflammatory drugs
PTH	parathyroid hormone
RBC	red blood cell
rt-PA	recombinant tissue-type plasminogen activator
SBP	systolic blood pressure
SD	standard deviation
SPECT	single photon emission computed tomography
SSRIs	selective serotonin reuptake inhibitors
T_3	triiodothyronine
T_4	thyroxine
TSH	thyroid-stimulating hormone
UA	urinalysis
UTI	urinary tract infection
WHI	Women's Health Initiative
WHO	World Health Organization

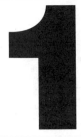

Approach to the Geriatric Patient: The Comprehensive Geriatric Assessment

Stanley J. Birge and
Steve R. Lai

PRINCIPLES OF GERIATRIC ASSESSMENT

Approach to the geriatric patient recognizes that functional disabilities and presenting complaints are a consequence of multiple factors, including medical, social, and environmental factors. In contrast to the assessment of a younger adult patient, **the geriatric assessment focuses on identifying functional deficits and developing recommendations either to correct those deficits or to modify the environment and social support systems to optimize the patient's independence.** Thus, the ideal geriatric assessment involves a team of multiple disciplines that includes, but is not limited to, a social worker, pharmacist, and physical therapist, in addition to the physician. **Studies have shown that a comprehensive geriatric assessment often leads to the identification of previously unrecognized medical and psychosocial problems and to more frequent medication changes, psychosocial evaluations, and use of community services.** Comprehensive multidisciplinary geriatric assessments are provided at most academic centers but are difficult to replicate in the private sector because of inadequate reimbursement.

This chapter provides a framework for the physician to assess elderly patients in a timely, cost-effective manner. The functional assessment tool in Fig. 1-1 exemplifies the type of evaluation that should be performed on all new patients >70 yrs or any patient with known deficits in instrumental activities of daily living (ADL). The functional assessment in the elderly is indicated not only to identify deficits in function but also to serve as a baseline to monitor changes in function that occur with treatment. In addition, numerous screening and assessment tools are conveniently provided in the Appendixes for rapid access when assessing elderly patients.

COGNITIVE FUNCTION

A discussion of the evaluation and management of dementia is provided in Chap. 3, Dementia. Assessment of the elderly patient is facilitated by the patient or caregiver completing a review of systems and a screen for dementia and depression before being seen by the physician [1]. **The essential element of the screen for dementia is the self-administered Clock Completion Test (CCT)** (see Appendix B). When combined with risk factors for dementia, the CCT provides better sensitivity and comparable specificity as the Short Blessed Test (SBT) (see Appendix A). A patient has an approximately 80% chance of having Alzheimer's disease if he or she has more or less than three numbers in the fourth clockwise quadrant. The CCT is also a useful instrument for assessing cognitive function in hospitalized patients with suspected delirium (see Chap. 4, Delirium).

The modified SBT (mSBT; see Appendix A) [2] is a recommended component of a geriatric assessment, even in the presence of a normal CCT, because the CCT is relatively insensitive in identifying patients with vascular dementia. Furthermore, an abnormal CCT does not provide information as to the severity of the dementia. The time required to recite the months of the year in reverse order (item five of the mSBT) provides an assessment of executive function that is sensitive to cerebral vascular insufficiency.

Patient's Name: _____ DOB: _____ Date: _____

Activities of daily living   Partial   Heavy   Has the Help
               Independent   Assist   Assist   Needed
Dressing   _____
Eating   _____
Bathing   _____
Toileting   _____
Transfers   _____
Instrumental activities of daily living
Meal preparation   _____
Shopping   _____
Medications   _____
Transportation   _____
Finances   _____

Lower extremity strength, gait, and balance
Stands up from chair: No ___ Yes ___, With ___ Without hands ___,
Time to do 5 ___ sec
Steps in 12 ft ___ Steps for turn ___ Time ___ sec, With ___ Without ___ assistive device
Steps in 12 ft ___ Steps for turn ___ Time ___ sec (distracted)
Progressive Romberg Score ____   Eyes open   Eyes closed
               Romberg stance   _____   _____
               Semi-tandem stance_____   _____
               Tandem stance   _____   _____

Vision: Reads newsprint without ___ with glasses ___
Hearing: Hears normal conversation without ___ with ___ hearing aid

Nutrition
           At age 50   Reported Current   Actual Current
   Weight   _____   _____   _____
   Height   _____   _____   _____
   Loss of 10 or more lbs in last 6 months Yes ___ No ___
   Dentition: adequate for chewing Yes ___ No ___, Denture Yes ___ No ___, Fit Yes ___ No ___

Depression
   During the past month, have you often been bothered by feeling down, depressed, or
hopeless? Yes ___ No ___
   During the past month, have you often been bothered by little interest or pleasure in
doing things? Yes ___ No ___

Washington University   Older Adult   Assessment   Program

FIG. 1-1. Geriatric assessment screen.

ACTIVITIES OF DAILY LIVING

The assessment of the ability to perform ADL is an abbreviated form of the Lawton and Katz ADL/instrumental ADL scales that is useful in identifying deficits that threaten independence but also for monitoring patients during treatment. The complete versions of these scales are provided in the Appendixes M and N.

STRENGTH, GAIT, AND BALANCE

Assessment of lower-extremity strength, gait, and balance is a sensitive predictor of independence and provides a quantitative measure of change in evaluating response to therapy. If the patient is able to stand from a sitting position with his or her arms folded across the chest; the patient is then asked to repeat the task five times as fast as he or she can. The time to do so correlates highly with more sophisticated measures, such as the Cybex dynamometer [3]. Times >10 secs suggest the presence of lower-extremity proximal muscle weakness. **Gait is assessed by asking the patient to walk 12 ft at his or her normal pace, turn, and return without stopping.** The number of steps required to traverse 12 ft and the number of steps required to turn 180 degrees provide a quantitative measure of dynamic balance. The task can be repeated with the distraction of counting backward from 20 while the patient walks. The disparity between the times of the two gait assessments is a measure of the patient's risk of falls. **The Progressive Romberg is a quantitative measure of static balance** [4]. The patient is asked to stand for 10 secs with his or her eyes open and then closed in three different positions: feet together (Romberg stance), one foot halfway in front of the other (semi-tandem stance), and the heel of one foot against the toe of the other (tandem stance). The score is the number of stances successfully maintained for 10 secs.

VISION

Vision can be screened with a Rosenbaum vision card (see Appendix J), or have the patient read the print on the assessment form with and without glasses (see Chap. 19, Ophthalmology and Geriatrics).

HEARING

Hearing can be screened by the Hearing Handicap Inventory in the Elderly or the Whisper Test (see Appendix K). Report the patient's ability to hear normal conversation with and without hearing aids.

NUTRITION

Nutritional assessment is critical because of the impact of protein-calorie and micronutrient deficiency on function. 15% of older outpatients and almost one-half of hospitalized elderly patients are malnourished. Poor nutrition leads to prolonged hospital stays, readmissions, pressure ulcers, and increased mortality. **There are often multiple factors related to malnutrition, including poverty, social isolation, depression, dementia, pain, immobility, reflux, constipation, alcoholism, medications, dental problems, and altered hunger and thirst recognition.** In addition, **dysphagia** due to strokes, parkinsonism, medicines, or dementia has been estimated to affect one-half of the institutionalized elderly population. Evidence of weight loss (>10 lbs in the past 6 mos) should prompt a lab assessment of the serum albumin, RBC indices, and total lymphocytes (see Chap. 9, Unintentional Weight Loss in the Elderly). **Vitamin D deficiency and resistance play a prominent role in falls and hip fracture** and may be suggested by a loss of height >2 in. A serum 25-hydroxyvitamin D measurement can confirm vitamin D deficiency. However, an elevated intact parathyroid hormone assay in patients with normal levels of serum calcium and 25-hydroxyvitamin D on >600-mg calcium diet is suggestive of vitamin D resistance. Zinc deficiency also plays a prominent role in geriatric syndromes, including immune deficiency, impaired wound healing, cognitive dysfunction, and sarcopenia. Because the major source of dietary zinc is red meat, assessment of dentition and dentures provides a simple approach to the screening for this problem. There is no reliable blood test for zinc deficiency. Appendix F includes an appetite and nutrition screening tool.

DEPRESSION

Unrecognized depression is common in the geriatric patient and is associated with a three- to fourfold increased risk of functional disability, Alzheimer's disease, and cardiovascular disease (see Chap. 5, Depression in the Older Adult). **Two screening questions identify 80% to 95% of adults affected by major depression** [5] (Fig. 1-1). Those with a positive response to one question should be evaluated by the Geriatric Depression Scale (see Appendix C) to ascertain the number of symptoms endorsed by the patient. **Patients with multiple symptoms who do not meet criteria for major depression have comparable outcomes to those who do and therefore should be treated.**

POLYPHARMACY

In long-term care facilities, the average resident takes seven different medications. Older patients often have numerous physicians and pharmacies. The initial step in assessing polypharmacy is to identify all prescription and over-the-counter drugs (see Chap. 6, Approach to Polypharmacy and Appropriate Medication Use). The clinician should write down all drugs by generic name and eliminate all unnecessary medications. Physicians must be aware of the age-related changes in drug metabolism. In the elderly, there are changes in body composition, liver and kidney metabolism, and pharmacodynamics. **Before a new drug is started, the clinician should identify risk factors for adverse drug reactions, such as advanced age, liver or kidney disease, or multiple medications.** Physicians can focus on improving compliance by keeping regimens simple and timing administration with meals.

CONTINENCE

It is estimated that 15–30% of community-dwelling older adults suffer from urinary incontinence, and almost 50% of older nursing home residents are affected (see Chap. 24, Urinary Incontinence). Elderly women are twice as likely to have urinary incontinence as elderly men. This increased prevalence is related to anatomic differences, pelvic floor dysfunction, and perineal injury. Incontinence in older men is usually related to prostatic enlargement and sphincter impairment. Additional factors contributing to urinary incontinence include UTI, confusional states, medication, immobility, hyperglycemia, alcohol abuse, congestive heart failure, catheter-induced bladder dysfunction, and stool impaction. **Physicians need to directly ask about urinary incontinence, as patients often do not openly admit to incontinence.** Patients need to be aware that most urinary incontinence problems can be evaluated with minimal testing and that most treatment options are nonsurgical.

MOTOR VEHICLE ACCIDENTS

Drivers aged >70 yrs have more accidents, more hospitalizations resulting from accidents, and more fatalities resulting from accidents than middle-aged drivers. The main factors contributing to impaired driving ability include a decline in visual acuity, hearing, information processing, and psychomotor skills. Because multiple domains of cognitive function contribute to impaired driving, no simple algorithm or test has been developed to reliably identify when a driver becomes unsafe (see Chap. 11, The Older Adult Driver).

SUGGESTED READING

Fleming KC, Evans JM, Weber DC, et al. Practical functional assessment of elderly persons: a primary care approach. *Mayo Clin Proc* 1995;70:890–910.

Goldberg TH, Chavin SI. Preventive medicine and screening in older adults. *J Am Geriatr Soc* 1997;45:344–354.

Lawton MP, Brody EM. Assessment of older people: self-maintaining and instrumental activities of daily living. *Gerontologist* 1969;9:179–186.

Scheitel SM, Fleming KC, Chutka DS, et al. Geriatric health maintenance. *Mayo Clin Proc* 1996;71:289–302.

REFERENCES

1. Ball LJ, Ogden A, Mandi D, et al. The validation of a mailed health survey for screening of dementia of the Alzheimer's type. *J Am Geriatr Soc* 2001;49:798–802.
2. Ball LJ, Bisher GB, Birge SJ. A simple test of central processing speed: an extension of the Short Blessed Test. *J Am Geriatr Soc* 1999;47:1359–1363.
3. Csuka M, McCarty DJ. Simple method for measurement of lower extremity muscle strength. *Am J Med* 1985;78:77–81.
4. Guralnik JM, Simonsick EM, Ferrucci L, et al. A short physical performance battery assess lower extremity function: association with self-reported disability and prediction of mortality and nursing home admission. *J Gerontol Med Sci* 1998; 49:M85–M94.
5. Whooley MA, Avins AL, Miranda J, et al. Case-finding instruments for depression: two questions are as good as many. *J Gen Intern Med* 1997;12:439–445.

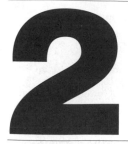

Settings for Geriatric Care

Kellie L. Flood

INTRODUCTION

For several years, the trend in health care has been toward shortened lengths of stay in the hospitalized setting and increasing care being delivered in the home or other venues. There has also been a growing recognition of the risk for complications and functional decline in older patients during a hospitalization. Following is a summary of different levels of care available for older adults.

MEDICARE AND MEDICAID

Government health benefits are available for the elderly (Medicare) and a portion of people in poverty (Medicaid). Persons eligible for Social Security payments because of age or disability are eligible for Medicare. These benefits include **Hospital Insurance (Part A) and Supplemental Medical Insurance, which requires paying premiums (Part B).** >98% of elders qualify for Part A without cost. Part A covers the cost of hospital admissions (after a deductible) and home health charges. Part B covers physician fees and outpatient medical and surgical services; supplies; tests; medical equipment; and physical, occupational, and speech therapies. **Medicare does not provide coverage for long-term nursing home care.**

Medicaid's range of services is more extensive, often providing coverage for glasses, dental work, and outpatient prescription drugs. It also covers long-term nursing home care. Some states offer Medicaid services targeted at elderly at risk for nursing home placement, such as comprehensive health and social services modeled by the Program for All Inclusive Care for the Elderly (see below).

HOSPITAL SETTING: ACUTE CARE FOR THE ELDERLY UNITS

Patients aged >65 represent approximately 40% of all acute care admissions and nearly 50% of inpatient days of care. For frail elderly (those with chronic diseases or disability), a hospitalization frequently results in an overall decline in function. Geriatric syndromes that may account for this decline include delirium, pressure sores, malnutrition, polypharmacy, deconditioning, falls, and depression [1]. **On discharge, 25–35% of elderly patients have lost independent functioning in one or more of the basic activities of daily living (ADL) during a hospitalization.** This functional decline is associated with increased length of stay, higher costs, and increased risk of temporary or permanent institutionalization for patients who were able to live at home before admission [2]. Models of care for these frail older inpatients to prevent functional decline have been developed.

The most effective interventions to prevent functional decline address multiple domains of health (functional, cognitive, psychosocial, medical). This model of care is implemented on **Acute Care for the Elderly (ACE) Units or Geriatric Evaluation and Management Units (GEMU).** These models use a patient-centered interdisciplinary approach to the care of hospitalized elderly patients. **This model of care is aimed at early recognition and prevention of geriatric syndromes.**

The model of care on an ACE Unit is to address all relevant disorders and geriatric syndromes, not just the admitting diagnosis. An ACE Unit consists of the following components [2,3]:

- Environmental modifications encouraging socialization, minimizing the use of restraints, and reducing the incidence of and risk for falls
- Patient-centered care emphasizing independence
- Nurse-initiated prevention protocols targeted at geriatric syndromes such as immobility and pressure sores, functional decline, incontinence, malnutrition, falls, depression, and delirium
- Frequent interdisciplinary team rounds reviewing functional status and monitoring for risk factors for decline, iatrogenic complications, and the development of geriatric syndromes
- Discharge planning from the day of admission

Several randomized clinical trials of ACE Units demonstrate improved outcomes in elderly patients admitted to a geriatric unit. These outcomes include better functional and mobility performance at discharge, greater improvement in ADL scores, fewer nursing home admissions at discharge, and lower charges compared to similar patients admitted to a general medicine floor [4–6]. There are conflicting data regarding the effect on length of stay [7–9]. A more recent study of a GEMU looking at mortality as the primary outcome in patients aged $\geq$ 75 yrs and meeting criteria for frailty demonstrated a >50% reduction in mortality at 3 mos that persisted to 6 mos (45% reduction) compared to usual medical care [7]. **This provides further evidence that the ACE Unit model of care should be the standard of care for all frail elderly admitted to a hospital.**

SUBACUTE CARE

At the time of discharge from a hospitalization, some older patients may still require a level of care or a need for rehabilitation that no longer warrants an inpatient admission but cannot be provided in the home setting. With the growing trend of reduced lengths of inpatient stays, a need has evolved for a level of care between hospitalization and home. This level of care is provided through subacute units (also referred to as **restorative care, skilled nursing facilities, intensive therapeutic care, transitional care, extended care,** etc.) These subacute units may be associated with a hospital or may be freestanding facilities. **The goal is to transition patients to a lower level of care such as discharge to home with or without home care services or assisted living.**

Eligibility is defined by the need for daily (5 days/wk) skilled nursing or rehabilitation services. These services include IV medications, enteral tube feedings, wound care, dressing changes, and physical and occupational therapy when there is a reasonable expectation for the patient's condition to improve. Some programs also provide chemotherapy, dialysis, total parenteral nutrition, and ventilator support.

Under the Medicare Skilled Nursing Facility Benefit, Medicare Part A recipients are eligible for up to 100 days of skilled nursing care or skilled rehabilitation services after a hospitalization of at least 3 days. Patients receive 100% coverage for the first 20 days and 80% coverage for the last 80 days. However, most Medicare supplements and Medicaid cover this copayment.

LONG-TERM CARE SETTINGS

Long-term care can be provided in a variety of settings, including in the home with supportive services and/or adult day health centers, assisted living facilities (ALFs), nursing homes, or newer models of care such as the Program for All-Inclusive Care for the Elderly (PACE).

Assisted Living

There is no uniform definition of what "assisted living" entails. In general, ALFs have been established as an alternative to nursing home placement for older adults who are no longer able to live independently but do not yet require total nursing care. These facilities may also be termed *residential care, adult congregate care,* or *community res-*

idential facilities. As of 1998, there were >11,000 ALFs in the United States, housing >500,000 residents. **These facilities encourage self-reliance by providing supportive services as needed in the resident's living environment as long as possible.** However, each facility varies in terms of its size, services provided, staffing, accommodations, and price. Most, but not all, ALFs offer at least a basic level of service that includes 24-hr staff oversight, housekeeping services, two or more meals a day, and personal assistance, which often includes reminders to take medications and assistance with ADL such as bathing and dressing. Other services offered may include home health care, physical and occupational therapies and nursing care (either provided by staff or through an agency), and recreation areas. Approximately 70% of facilities have a licensed nurse on staff; however, approximately 20% of facilities do not provide any monitoring of care by a licensed nurse. Many facilities also provide recreation areas and structured activities designed to promote socialization and prevent isolation.

The housing accommodations may take the form of a private or semiprivate room in a facility or a freestanding apartment in a complex. These complexes may also provide tiered levels of care ranging from independent living to nursing home care. **This may provide for ease of transition as a resident's care needs change over time.**

Eligibility criteria vary from site to site. In a 1998 national survey, up to 40% of ALFs would admit residents with cognitive impairment. However, **most will exclude residents with severe impairment or behavioral problems or cases in which concerns for safety exist** (such as wandering or leaving on stove burners). Also, up to 60% of the facilities surveyed would accept residents with moderate physical limitations requiring use of a wheelchair or walker. However, most would not admit patients with limitations that required assistance with transfers. **Many sites require that the resident is able to negotiate a path to safety in case of fire.**

Assisted living is *not covered by Medicare or Medicaid* and is largely not affordable for low- or moderate-income persons. However, Medicaid recipients in some states may receive a stipend to help defray the cost.

Program for All-Inclusive Care for the Elderly

PACE is a capitated Medicare and Medicaid managed care program that integrates the delivery of acute and long-term care to frail older adults in the community. PACE has >25 sites across the United States. The primary goal is to enable frail elders who meet qualifications for nursing home placement to continue to live in the community by providing comprehensive care that addresses medical, psychosocial, and functional needs. To qualify for enrollment, a person must be ≥ 55 yrs, live in the catchment area defined by that PACE program, and be eligible for nursing home care as determined by the state's Medicaid criteria. The enrollee must also demonstrate the ability to live safely at home when not at the PACE center. **The typical PACE center is a freestanding adult health center (including a pharmacy and recreational, physical, and occupational therapy areas) with a full-service medical clinic.** PACE services are provided at the site as well as in the home or any inpatient facilities, including nursing homes.

Care is provided by an interdisciplinary team consisting of primary care physicians, nurse practitioners, clinic nurses, home health nurses, social workers, occupational and physical therapists, dietitians, recreational therapists, and spiritual care staff. **Transportation is provided** between the center and home or off-site medical appointments. Care plans are created by the interdisciplinary team and are reviewed quarterly at team meetings. Enrollees are transported to the center 5–7 days/wk, based on need and the care plan. Goals of the PACE program include the following:

* Prevent unnecessary hospitalizations and premature institutionalization
* Provide quality and cost-effective comprehensive care to frail elders
* Provide acute and long-term care by a single organization, easing communication among providers and using an interdisciplinary approach

PACE provides this full range of services for the lifetime of the enrollee in exchange for a fixed monthly payment from Medicare and Medicaid. Waivers are granted to

PACE programs by Medicare and Medicaid, allowing more extensive services than those provided by standard benefits. Patients who are not eligible to receive Medicaid must pay out-of-pocket for that portion of the fees. Otherwise, PACE enrollees pay no additional fees or copayments for any service. There is no cap on service use. Enrollees must receive primary care and services from PACE physicians and staff. Although assuming financial risk for cost overruns, thus far PACE programs remain financially viable. This program has met with national success, providing quality of care that rivals or exceeds traditional fee-for-service Medicare, and has low disenrollment rates.

Nursing Home Care

As of 1993, payment by Medicare to nursing homes exceeded $223 billion, approximately 25% of total healthcare expenditures. >1.5 million Americans reside in nursing homes. However, rates of nursing home admissions have declined slightly as alternative avenues of care and home services have become more prevalent. In 1997, only 11/1,000 persons aged 65–74 yrs resided in a nursing home, compared with 46/1,000 persons aged 75–84 yrs and 192/1,000 persons aged 85 yrs and older. Despite the use of newer community-based services to the frail older adult, the total number of nursing home residents is only expected to rise as the population continues to age. Also, the percentage of nursing home residents with functional limitations has increased.

Timely assessments in several disciplines are recommended for optimal care of nursing home residents. **Patients admitted to a nursing home must receive a physician assessment within 48–72 hrs of admission and then subsequently every 30–60 days.** This physician may be an assigned nursing home physician or the patient's private practitioner. **A copy of the patient's entire record from a hospitalization and any recommendations and physician orders should accompany the patient to the nursing home.** These orders may include frequency of vital signs; lab tests; scheduled radiographic studies; need for therapies such as physical, occupational, or speech therapy; wound care; diet; and precaution orders to prevent aspiration or falls. A licensed nurse assesses each resident on the day of admission and daily thereafter. The extent of involvement of other disciplines in the assessment and care-planning processes varies depending on the resident's problems, the availability of various professionals, and state and federal regulations. **The interdisciplinary team involved in the development and implementation of a resident's care plan should include representatives from nursing, social services, nutrition, and rehabilitation.** See Appendix P for more information on Selected Topics and Useful Resources for Older Adults.

KEY POINTS TO REMEMBER

- The current trend in health care has shifted toward shortened lengths of stay in the hospitalized setting and care being delivered increasingly in the home or other venues.
- Hospitalization of the frail elderly frequently results in potentially preventable decline in overall function.
- Specialized geriatric inpatient units have been developed for the frail elderly that have been shown to reduce decline in ADL, decrease length of stay, decrease rates of institutionalization, and reduce mortality.
- The goal of subacute care is to transition patients from the hospital to a lower level of care such as discharge to home with or without home care services or assisted living.
- The care and services provided by ALFs are varied, but generally entail relatively independent living with the availability of some assistance with ADL, medication administration, skilled therapy, 24-hr staff oversight, and opportunities for socialization.
- Most ALFs require that the patient can negotiate a path to safety.

SUGGESTED READING

Eleazer PG. The challenge of measuring quality of care in PACE. Program of All Inclusive Care for the Elderly. *J Am Geriatr Soc* 2000;48:1019–1020.

Eng C, Pedulla J, Eleazer GP, et al. Program of All-inclusive Care for the Elderly (PACE): an innovative model of integrated geriatric care and financing. *J Am Geriatr Soc* 1997;45(2):223.

Federal Interagency Forum on Aging-Related Statistics. Older Americans 2000: key indicators of well-being. Available at: http://www.agingstats.gov. Accessed April 2003.

Hawes C, Rose M, Phillips OS. A national study of assisted living for the frail elderly: Results of a National Survey of Facilities, 3. Available at: http://aspe.os.dhhs.gov/daltcp/reports/facreses.htm. Accessed April 2003.

Hazard WR, Ouslander JG, Blass JP, et al., eds. *Principles of geriatric medicine and gerontology*, 4th ed. New York: McGraw-Hill, 1999.

REFERENCES

1. Palmer RM, Counsell S, Landefeld CS. Clinical intervention trials: the ACE unit. *Acute Hosp Care* 1998;14(4):831.
2. Lyons WL, Landefeld CS. Improving care for hospitalized elders. *Ann Long Term Care* 2001;9(4):35.
3. Kresevic D, Counsell SR, Covinsky K, et al. A patient-centered model of acute care for elders. *Nurs Clin North Am* 1998;33(3):515.
4. Collard AF, Bachman SS, Beatrice DF. Acute care delivery for the geriatric patient: an innovative approach. *QRB Qual Rev Bull* 1985;11(6):180.
5. Boyer N, Chuang JL, Gipner D. An acute care geriatric unit. *Nurs Manag* 1986;17(5):22.
6. Rubenstein LZ, Josephson KR, Wieland GD, et al. Effectiveness of a geriatric evaluation unit. A randomized clinical trial. *N Engl J Med* 1984;311:1664.
7. Saltvedt I, Opdahl ES, Fayers P, et al. Reduced mortality in treating acutely sick, frail older patients in a geriatric evaluation and management unit. A prospective randomized trial. *J Am Geriatr Soc* 2002;50:792.
8. Saunders RH, Hickler RB, Hall SA, et al. A geriatric special-care unit: experience in a university hospital. *J Am Geriatr Soc* 1983;31:685.
9. Landefeld CS, Palmer RM, Kresevic D, et al. A randomized trial of care in a hospital medical unit especially designed to improve the functional outcomes of acutely ill older patients. *N Engl J Med* 1995;332:1338.

Dementia

Monique Williams
and Kyle C. Moylan

INTRODUCTION

Dementia is a syndrome defined by a progressive decline in multiple areas of cognitive functioning sufficient to interfere with social and occupational functioning. Dementia is further characterized as a decline in cognitive function from a previous level in an individual without clouded consciousness. **It is not a consequence of normal aging** but usually occurs late in life. Patients with dementia have memory impairment and at least one of the following: aphasia, apraxia, agnosia, or a decline in executive function. **Alzheimer's disease (AD)** is the single most common etiology of dementia and is the prototype for this discussion.

It is important to evaluate dementia and make a specific diagnosis (beyond ruling out reversible etiologies). Treatments are currently available for the symptoms of AD, and more will be available in the coming years. In addition, early recognition of a progressive neurologic process gives patients and families much-needed information about the expected course of their illness. It also facilitates end of life decision making and allows for financial and living arrangements to be made (Table 3-1).

Epidemiology

Dementia is the fourth leading cause of death in the United States. In ambulatory individuals aged 75–85 yrs, dementia occurs with the same frequency as myocardial infarction and more frequently than strokes.

The prevalence of dementia increases dramatically with age: approximately 10% at age 65 and 50% at age 85.

Dementia is a public health issue with profound societal impact. AD affects 4 million individuals in the United States at a cost of $100 million annually (primarily costs associated with long-term care). The emotional impact on family and caregivers is immeasurable.

CAUSES

Pathophysiology

The pathologic hallmarks of AD are **senile plaques and neurofibrillary tangles,** which essentially represent an imbalance between neuronal injury and repair. These pathologic changes are accompanied by losses of synaptic connections, neurons, and neurotransmitters. Brain areas affected include the entorhinal cortex, hippocampus, limbic lobes, and neocortex.

The primary components of neurofibrillary tangles are filaments of abnormally phosphorylated tau protein. Senile (neuritic) plaques are composed of abnormally processed beta-amyloid protein, degenerating neurons, and surrounding inflammatory cells. **Amyloid precursor protein** is a transmembrane protein that is normally cleaved by alpha secretase into the beta-amyloid protein. Gene mutations in the amyloid precursor protein and presenilin genes have been identified that result in increased production of neurotoxic amyloid 1-42, cleaved from amyloid precursor protein by gamma-secretase

TABLE 3-1. DEFINITION OF DEMENTIA

Dementia is defined as multiple cognitive deficits manifested as **memory impairment plus one or more of the following**[a]:

Aphasia: language disturbance (e.g., word finding difficulty)

Apraxia: inability to carry out motor activities despite intact motor function (e.g., dressing)

Agnosia: inability to recognize or identify objects despite intact sensory function

Disturbance in executive functioning (e.g., planning, organizing, sequencing, abstract thinking)

[a]Sufficient to interfere with social and occupational functioning.

activity. Early-onset, familial AD accounts for <10% of cases and may be inherited in an autosomal dominant pattern.

PRESENTATION

Clinical Features of Alzheimer's Disease

AD is the single most common cause of dementia, accounting for 65–75% of cases. It is anticipated that there will be 14 million individuals with AD in the United States by 2040.

Risk factors for AD include age, family history of AD or Down's syndrome, history of depression, previous head injury (with loss of consciousness), female gender, osteoporosis, cerebrovascular or cardiovascular disease, and the apoprotein E4 allele.

The onset of AD is insidious and can be difficult to recognize in the early stages.

AD manifests as the clinical triad of memory impairment, visuospatial defects, and language impairment. **The clinical course is always progressive** with the typical progression outlined in Table 3-2.

Difficulty performing activities of daily living (ADL) is a key feature, eventually leading to complete dependence.

As the disease progresses, behavioral changes occur. These include personality changes, agitation, impulsiveness, poor judgment, suspiciousness, apathy, and depression. Death usually ensues 8–10 yrs after symptom onset.

Clinical Characteristics of Other Types of Dementia

- **Many cases of dementia are multifactorial.** For example, approximately one-half of AD patients may also have coexisting vascular or Lewy body pathology. AD occurs commonly in older patients with Parkinson's disease (PD), with one-half of the patients meeting neuropathologic criteria for AD at autopsy.

- **Dementia with Lewy bodies (or diffuse Lewy body disease) is a recently recognized disorder that may be the second most common cause of dementia** (see Chap. 26, Parkinson's Disease and Related Disorders). Autopsy series indicate that Lewy body dementia accounts for 25% of dementia cases. There is some overlap with both AD and PD, and the nomenclature of these diagnoses is still evolving (dementia with Lewy bodies, PD with dementia, diffuse Lewy body disease, Lewy body variant of AD, etc.).
  - **Parkinsonian features** occur early in the course. Conversely, dementia occurs late in the course of idiopathic PD, and some parkinsonian features develop very late in the course of AD. Symmetric rigidity and bradykinesia with postural instability occur more commonly than tremor, usually within 1 yr of cognitive decline.
  - **Spontaneous visual hallucinations occur early in the course** and may be worsened by treatment with dopaminergic agents. Patients are very sensitive to neuroleptic agents, which can cause severe worsening of parkinsonism.

TABLE 3-2. CLINICAL COURSE OF ALZHEIMER'S DISEASE

Early dementia	Moderate dementia	Advanced dementia
Reduction in productive and spontaneous activities	Reduced cognitive function	Remnants of memory remain
	More dependent in activities	Communication is limited to repeated words
Impairment in cognition		Eventual mutism
Reduced verbal output	Long-term memory altered	Bladder and bowel incontinence
Inability to cope with complex or new tasks	Further decline in verbal output	Complete assistance with daily activities
Retention of well-learned behavior	Behavioral changes: wandering, hostility, verbal outbursts, aggression, and psychosis	Death due to sepsis, pneumonia, pulmonary embolus, or other illnesses associated with immobility
Misplacing items without independent retrieval		
Problems with financial matters	Independent living is dangerous	
Difficulties with visuo-spatial organization		
Decreased initiative, depression, restlessness, overactivity		

- **Other key features include slowing of thought and actions** (bradyphrenia and psychomotor slowing).
- **Repeated falls** are common early in the course.
- **The symptoms tend to fluctuate,** with some episodes of clouded consciousness mimicking delirium.
- Dementia with Lewy bodies is treated with dopaminergic agents, as with PD, but the response tends to be less favorable. Cholinesterase inhibitors may also be effective for the cognitive symptoms with a small risk of worsening the parkinsonism.

- PD is frequently associated with dementia and is discussed in detail in Chap. 26, Parkinson's Disease and Related Disorders.

- **Vascular dementia (multiinfarct dementia)** is perhaps the most controversial dementia diagnosis; pure vascular dementia is probably uncommon. Cerebrovascular accidents can complicate the course of dementia of any type. Discrete areas of cerebral infarction occur in AD patients and may correlate with the severity of cognitive dysfunction [1]. The majority of patients who carry the diagnosis of vascular dementia have plaques and tangles at autopsy, in part because **there are no well-accepted diagnostic criteria.** In addition, cerebrovascular disease may trigger or accelerate the expression of AD:
  - The clinical course demonstrates **a stepwise deterioration** in function, as opposed to the relentless progression of AD.
  - Patients may have traditional **vascular risk factors,** including HTN, diabetes, hyperlipidemia, smoking, coronary artery disease, and cerebrovascular disease.
  - **Common features** include urinary dysfunction, gait disturbances, and loss of executive function. Focal neurologic signs may be present, including cortical motor and sensory deficits or abnormal reflexes.
  - **Treatment focuses on treating vascular risk factors** (antiplatelet therapy, cholesterol lowering, tobacco cessation, BP control, etc.), but cholinesterase inhibitors may also be beneficial (see below). Some patients may exhibit worsening cognitive function with lower BPs (<130/80). ACE inhibitors are preferred

agents, but the use of any antihypertensive agent warrants the close monitoring of cognitive function.

• **Frontotemporal dementia (e.g., Pick's disease)** is typified by disordered executive function (initiation and planning) and disinhibited behavior (labile affect and sexual inappropriateness). Language dysfunction is also prominent, with a progressive reduction in speech, stereotypy, echolalia, and perseveration. Cognitive dysfunction is usually mild with relative preservation of visuospatial orientation and praxias.

• **Creutzfeldt-Jacob disease** is a prion disease characterized by a rapidly progressive course (death in <1 yr), myoclonus, cerebellar dysfunction, and characteristic EEG findings. It is rare in the United States but important to recognize. Diagnosis is confirmed by brain biopsy.

• **Normal pressure hydrocephalus** is marked by the clinical triad of gait disorder, urinary incontinence, and cognitive decline (usually in that order). Unfortunately, these findings are common in many patients with dementia. The gait disturbance is characterized by gait apraxia. Focal cortical signs and psychosis are rare. Cognitive disturbances include **psychomotor slowing, impaired concentration, and mild memory impairment.** CT may suggest the diagnosis if enlarged ventricles are present, but radionucleotide studies and the Miller-Fisher test help confirm the diagnosis. Treatment involves placement of a **ventriculoperitoneal shunt,** which is not always effective.

EVALUATION

Timely evaluation and diagnosis of dementia is essential for effective management of the patient and requires symptomatic screening.
Dementia is a diagnosis of inclusion, based on information obtained from the history, physical exam, and cognitive testing.
Most cases of dementia are initially seen in primary care settings. It is essential that primary care physicians are familiar with the various forms of dementia and their evaluation. With appropriate diagnostic tools, clinical diagnostic accuracy can exceed 90%.
Mild cognitive impairment (MCI) is a heterogeneous clinical entity, including individuals who are at the low-normal spectrum of normal aging; those who have benign, nonprogressive MCI; and a subset who progress to dementia. Patients with MCI have subjective and objective evidence of impaired cognition, which represents a decline from baseline but does not meet criteria for dementia. Patients with MCI are at increased risk of developing dementia [2,3].
Referral to a neurologist is appropriate in cases with **atypical features,** including onset at <60 yrs, rapidly progressive course, or significant abnormalities on neurologic exam (motor abnormalities, abnormal reflexes, cerebellar signs).

History

The history should be obtained from the patient and a reliable collateral source. The informant should be someone who knows the patient well and has frequent interactions.
The interview should focus on the following:

• The nature of symptom onset (insidious vs. sudden)
• The duration of symptoms
• Characteristics of progression (gradual vs. stepwise deterioration)
• Areas of impairment (recognition of people, geographic and temporal disorientation, remembering appointments and medications, language impairment)
• The presence of hallucinations, suspicions, or delusions
• Extent of impairment in instrumental ADL (managing finances, driving, using the telephone) and ADL (bathing, dressing, continence)

TABLE 3-3. MEDICATIONS THAT CAN CAUSE COGNITIVE DYSFUNCTION

Antiarrhythmic agents	Histamine receptor blockers
Antibiotics	Immunosuppressive agents
Anticholinergic agents	Muscle relaxants
Anticonvulsants	Narcotic analgesics
Tricyclic antidepressants	Sedative/hypnotics
Antiemetics	Antihypertensive agents
Antihistamines/decongestants	Antiparkinsonian agents

- Information pertaining to the patient's living situation, caregivers, and other sources of support
- Alcohol consumption
- Changes in mood and personality
- Family history
- Medications that could impair cognition (Table 3-3)

The history is often the only way to distinguish AD from other disorders that can disturb cognition (Table 3-4). **Depression and dementia frequently coexist in the same patient** [4] (see Chap. 5, Depression in the Older Adult). Depression is common in patients with dementia, who may present atypically by wandering, by crying out, with aggression, or with functional decline. The diagnosis can be difficult, because some neurovegetative symptoms may develop in uncomplicated dementia. **Depression itself can cause cognitive impairment (pseudodementia) that may be reversible.** Differentiating between the two scenarios can be difficult, and there is no way to accurately predict which patients treated with antidepressants will show cognitive improvement. Pseudodemented patients are more likely to complain of cognitive difficulties than patients with true dementia are. **Part of the evaluation of dementia should include a screen for depression (see Appendix C)** **Dementia must be distinguished from delirium** (see Chap. 4, Delirium). Delirium is characterized by fluctuations in level of consciousness, disorientation, and impairment in attention and concentration. It has abrupt onset and short duration, whereas dementia is a chronic, slowly progressive disorder with a normal level of consciousness.

TABLE 3-4. DIFFERENTIAL DIAGNOSIS OF COGNITIVE DYSFUNCTION

Neurologic diseases	Systemic processes
Alzheimer's disease	Metabolic disease (renal, hepatic)
Lewy body dementia	Vitamin B_{12} deficiency
Vascular dementia	Neurosyphilis
Frontal lobe dementia	Hypothyroidism or hyperthyroidism
Prion disease	Drugs
Parkinson's disease	Hypercalcemia
Huntington chorea	Depression (pseudodementia)
Brain tumor	Delirium
Subdural hematoma	HIV
Normal pressure hydrocephalus	Rheumatologic disease (cerebral vasculitis)
Encephalitis	Hypovitaminosis D

Physical Exam and Cognitive Testing

A **complete physical and neurologic exam** should be performed. The neurologic exam is focused on alertness, motor function, parkinsonism, sensation, reflexes (including primitive reflexes), gait, and language. Physical signs of hypothyroidism to note include hypothermia, delayed relaxation of deep tendon reflexes, and myxedema.

A **mental status exam**, such as the modified Short Blessed Test, should be administered. (See Appendix A). A score of >8/28 on the Short Blessed Test is consistent with dementia.

The time required to recite the months of the year in reverse order (item five of the modified Short Blessed Test) provides an assessment of executive function that is sensitive to cerebral vascular insufficiency [5]. It can be used to monitor the initiation of antihypertensive therapy. Prolongation of the time from baseline would suggest inadequate cerebral perfusion and the need to allow the BP to rise.

Clock drawing (Clock Completion Test; see Appendix B) is a quick test that assesses memory, executive function, and visual construction skills and has excellent sensitivity and specificity for cognitive impairment. When combined with risk factors for dementia, the Clock Completion Test provides better sensitivity and comparable specificity as the MMSE or Short Blessed Test. A patient has an approximately 80% chance of having AD if they have > or <3 numbers in the fourth clockwise quadrant [6]. The Clock Completion Test is also a useful instrument for rapidly assessing cognitive function in hospitalized patients with suspected delirium (see Chap. 4, Delirium).

For patients with MCI or a high level of cognitive functioning, more extensive neuropsychometric testing may be required for diagnosis and monitoring progression. The clinical history may be the only evidence of the diagnosis.

Diagnostic Studies

Lab evaluation includes CBCs, basic electrolytes, calcium, liver function tests, thyroid panel, vitamin B$_{12}$, and syphilis serologies. Other tests may be obtained as relevant to specific patients: HIV, toxicology, heavy metals screen, and evaluation for rheumatologic disorders. Apoprotein E4 testing is currently only useful in clinical research.

Neuroimaging should be considered in all patients with dementia of <1 yr's duration but is not necessary for most cases. A noncontrast head CT is usually sufficient to screen for normal pressure hydrocephalus, subdural hematoma, and cerebrovascular disease. MRI is more sensitive for detecting vascular pathology but is of limited use in distinguishing between different types of dementia in individual patients [7]. Functional imaging techniques, such as fMRI, SPECT, or PET scans, are still investigative tools not recommended for routine clinical use.

MANAGEMENT

The management of dementia is predominately nonpharmacologic. Some nonpharmacologic strategies for improving function and behavior are listed in Table 3-5.

The first step is to establish a specific diagnosis.

The second step is to **empower the patient and his or her caregivers with information.** They need to understand what the diagnosis means, how it was made, and what the implications are. Frequently, just understanding the process is a relief to caregivers.

Participation in caregiver support groups and educational programs can improve caregiver satisfaction and delay institutionalization. The Alzheimer's Association is an invaluable resource for patients with dementia of any type. Local chapters offer classes about dementia and aspects of caregiving, as well as coping strategies for family and respite services. Resources vary by location, but most geriatric physicians should be familiar with the available organizations and assistance.

The **living arrangements** need to be addressed (see Chap. 2, Settings for Geriatric Care) and plans made for future needs.

The patient's **ability to drive** should be discussed (see Chap. 11, The Older Adult Driver). Patients with early dementia may be able to drive after a more formal driving

**TABLE 3-5. STRATEGIES TO IMPROVE FUNCTIONAL PERFORMANCE
AND REDUCE PROBLEM BEHAVIORS IN PATIENTS WITH DEMENTIA**

Strategy	Strength of evidence
To improve functional performance	
Behavior modification, scheduled toileting, prompted voiding to reduce urinary incontinence	Strong
Graded assistance, practice, and positive reinforcement to increase functional independence	Good
Low lighting levels, music, and simulated nature sounds to improve eating behaviors	Weak
Intensive multimodality group training to improve activities of daily living	Weak
To reduce problem behaviors	
Music, particularly during meals and bathing	Good
Walking or other forms of light exercise	Good
Simulated presence therapy, such as use of videotapes of family	Weak
Massage	Weak
Comprehensive psychosocial care programs	Weak
Pet therapy	Weak
Using commands issued at the patient's comprehension level	Weak
Bright light, white noise	Weak
Cognitive remediation	Weak

From American Academy of Neurology guideline summary for point of care: detection, diagnosis, and management of dementia. Available at: http://nucleus.con.ohio-state.edu/APN/ANP2/Neuro/md_summary.htm. Accessed April 2003, with permission.

assessment ensures that it is safe, whereas patients with more advanced dementia should not be allowed to drive.

If the patient has the capacity to make medical decisions, he or she should be encouraged to make arrangements such as advanced directives or a durable power of attorney. Patients without decision-making capacity need to have surrogate decision makers or a legal guardian appointed.

Treatment

Specific pharmacologic treatment for dementia is indicated to slow symptom progression, stabilize functional status, and delay institutionalization.

Cholinesterase inhibitors are currently the only drugs FDA approved for the treatment of AD. The most data are available supporting their use in patients with mild to moderate AD. They may be of some benefit in improving problem behaviors in patients with more advanced dementia or in delaying the development of dementia in patients with MCI. More data are also emerging regarding their efficacy for the treatment of vascular dementia [8], dementia with Lewy bodies [9], and other types of dementia.

Cholinesterase inhibitors do not alter the disease process but improve symptoms by enhancing cholinergic neurotransmission. Most patients show stabilization in the rate of cognitive decline, loss of ADL, and impairment of global function, typically lasting for several months [10–12]. Some patients may show temporary improvement in symptoms or no detectable response at all. The benefits of long-term treatment are less clear.

- Tacrine was the first cholinesterase inhibitor approved for use but is no longer used because of safer alternatives.
- **Donepezil** (Aricept) is convenient to use because of once-daily administration and efficacy at the starting dose. The initial dose is 5 mg PO daily, which is increased to 10 mg after 6 wks if tolerated. Giving the dose in the evening may minimize the effects on sleep.
- **Rivastigmine** (Exelon) has comparable efficacy to the other cholinesterase inhibitors. Disadvantages include more dose titration, more side effects at higher doses, and multiple daily (2–3) doses with food. The dose is titrated by 1.5-mg increments q2wks. The usual dose is 6–12 mg/day divided bid.
- **Galantamine** (Reminyl) has similar efficacy and has some interactions with presynaptic nicotinic receptors, the clinical effect of which is unknown. Initial dose is typically 4 mg PO bid. The usual dosage is 8–24 mg/day divided bid with food. The dose is titrated in 4-wk intervals.
- **Side effects** are similar for all cholinesterase inhibitors and include GI effects (nausea, diarrhea, anorexia), sleep disturbance, and behavior problems. **Dose titration over several weeks minimizes the side effects, which tend to improve with continued use.**
- **Contraindications** include hypersensitivity reactions and cardiac conduction defects (bradycardia, heart block). Concomitant use of anticholinergic medications should be avoided.
- **Assessing the benefit of treatment** in an individual patient is difficult, as the untreated course varies substantially from person to person. Discontinuing cholinesterase inhibitors, even when there has not been a detectable clinical benefit, can result in a decline in cognitive function. It is important that patients and caregivers understand these limitations.

Vitamin E is recommended for all patients to slow the progression of AD. One trial has demonstrated delayed time to nursing home placement, severe dementia, death, or loss of ability to perform ADL compared with placebo [13]. This difference was only significant after adjusting for differences in baseline Mini-Mental Status Exam scores, and no effect on cognitive testing was noted. The dose used in the study was 2000 IU qd, but most physicians recommend **400–800 IU PO qd.** There are no serious side effects, although it may potentiate the effects of warfarin and other anticoagulants.

Vascular risk factors should be identified and treated, particularly for those patients whose history and exam reveal abnormalities consistent with cerebrovascular disease (see Vascular dementia).

Depression is common in the patient with dementia and often leads to functional decline, weight loss, behavior disturbances, and reduced quality of life. Suspected depression should be treated appropriately (see Chap. 5, Depression in the Older Adult). Tricyclic antidepressants should be avoided because of possible adverse effects on cognitive function.

Agitated behaviors that do not respond to nonpharmacologic management and caregiver education may require specific pharmacologic treatment. Paranoia, delusions, hallucinations, and aggression are indications to consider adjunctive treatment with antipsychotic agents. Long-term use is associated with potential adverse effects, particularly drug-induced extrapyramidal effects. Atypical antipsychotics, such as risperidone (Risperdal), olanzapine (Zyprexa, Zyprexa Zydis), and quetiapine (Seroquel), are preferred to haloperidol (Haldol) and other older neuroleptics.

Follow-Up

Follow-up visits should focus on changes in behavior, mood, and cognitive abilities along with their effects on daily functioning. The appropriate level of supervision and care should be periodically reevaluated, with plans made for future needs. Psychotropic medications and their indications should also be monitored so that attempts can be made to minimize or eliminate their use. As the disease progresses, the needs of caregivers become increasingly important, with the goal of delaying or preventing nursing home placement.

KEY POINTS TO REMEMBER

- Dementia is a syndrome defined by a progressive decline in multiple areas of cognitive functioning sufficient to interfere with social and occupational functioning.
- AD is the most common single cause of dementia.
- AD is characterized by an insidious onset and progressive course with loss of memory and other cognitive capabilities.
- Diffuse Lewy body disease is characterized by subcortical dementia, parkinsonism, visual hallucinations, fluctuating course, and early falls.
- Cerebrovascular disease can cause dementia alone or along with other entities. Treatment of vascular risk factors is indicated to slow disease progression.
- Frontotemporal dementia is characterized by disordered executive function, personality changes, disinhibited behavior, and language problems.
- MCI describes patients with evidence of cognitive decline without dementia, many of whom will progress to dementia.
- The diagnosis of dementia and AD is made primarily on clinical grounds, based on the collateral history supported by neuropsychometric testing.
- Successful management of dementia uses nonpharmacologic interventions to educate patients and caregivers, reducing caregiver burden.
- Cholinesterase inhibitors are effective at slowing clinical progression in patients with dementia of varying types and stages. Efficacy and side effects are similar with the three commonly used agents—donepezil, rivastigmine, and galantamine.
- Goals of cholinesterase inhibitor therapy include preservation of cognitive abilities and ability to perform ADL, while reducing caregiver burden and delaying institutionalization. They do not treat the underlying pathology.
- Most patients with dementia should be advised to take supplemental vitamin E.

SUGGESTED READING

Alzheimer A. Über eine eigenartige Erkrankung der Hirnrinde. *Allg Z Psychiatr Psych Geriat Med* 1907;64:146–148.

American Academy of Neurology guideline summary for point of care: detection, diagnosis, and management of dementia. Available at: http://nucleus.con.ohio-state.edu/APN/ANP2/Neuro/md_summary.htm. Accessed April 2003.

American Psychiatric Association. *Diagnostic and statistical manual of mental disorders*, 4th ed. Washington, DC: American Psychiatric Association, 1994.

Birge S. Practical strategies for the diagnosis and management of Alzheimer's disease. 1999;7:56–74.

Brown FW. Late-life psychosis: making the diagnosis and controlling symptoms. *Geriatrics* 1998;53:26–42.

Bullock R. New drugs for Alzheimer's disease and other dementias. *Br J Psychiatry* 2002;180:135–139.

Carlson DL, Fleming KC, Smith GE, et al. Management of dementia-related behavioral disturbances: a nonpharmacologic approach. *Mayo Clin Proc* 1995;70:1108–1115.

Cummings JL, Vinters HV, Cole GM, et al. Alzheimer's disease: etiologies, pathophysiology, cognitive reserve, and treatment opportunities. *Neurology* 1998;51(Suppl 1):S2–S17.

Fleming KC, Adams A, Peterson RC. Dementia: diagnosis and evaluation. *Mayo Clin Proc* 1995;70:1093–1107.

Hansen L, Salmon D, Galasko D, et al. The Lewy body variant of Alzheimer's disease: a clinical and pathological entity. *Neurology* 1990;40:1–8.

Lapalio LR, Sakla SS. Distinguishing Lewy body dementia. *Hosp Pract* 1998;33:93–108.

Martin JB. Molecular basis of the neurodegenerative disorders. *N Engl J Med* 1999;340:1970–1980.

Mayeux R, Sano M. Treatment of Alzheimer's disease. *N Engl J Med* 1999;341:1670–1679.

McKeith IG. Dementia with Lewy bodies. *Br J Psychiatry* 2002;180:144–147.

McKeith IG, Galasko D, Kosaka K, et al. Consensus guidelines for the clinical and pathologic diagnosis of dementia with Lewy bodies (DLB): report of the consortium on DLB international workshop. *Neurology* 1996;47:1113–1124.

Morris JC. The nosology of dementia. *Neurol Clin* 2000;18:773–788.

Morris JC, Storandt M, Miller JP, et al. Mild cognitive impairment represents early-stage Alzheimer disease. *Arch Neurol* 2001;58:397–405.

Small GW, Rabins PV, Barry PP, et al. Diagnosis and treatment of Alzheimer's disease and related disorders: consensus statement of the American Association for Geriatric Psychiatry, the Alzheimer's Association, and the American Geriatrics Society. *JAMA* 1997;278:1363–1371.

Snowden JS, Neary D, Mann DM. Frontotemporal dementia. *Br J Psychiatry* 2002; 180:140–143.

REFERENCES

1. Snowden JS, Greiner LH, Mortimer JA, et al. Brain infarction and the clinical expression of Alzheimer's disease: the nun study. *JAMA* 1997;277:813–817.
2. Peterson RC, Stevens JC, Ganguli M, et al. Practice parameter: early detection of dementia: mild cognitive impairment (an evidence-based review). *Neurology* 2001;56:1133–1142.
3. Galvin JE, Lee VM, Trojanowski JQ. Synucleinopathies: clinical and pathological implications. *Arch Neurol* 2001;58:186–190.
4. Migliorelli R, Teson A, Sabe L, et al. Prevalence and correlates of dysthymia and major depression among patients with Alzheimer's disease. *Am J Psychiatry* 1995;152:37–44.
5. Ball LJ, Bisher GB, Birge SJ. A simple test of central processing speed: an extension of the Short Blessed Test. *J Am Geriatr Soc* 1999;47:1359–1363.
6. Watson YI, Arfken CL, Birge SJ. Clock completion: an objective screening test for dementia. *J Am Geriatr Soc* 1993;41:1235–1240.
7. Varma AR, Laitt R, Lloyd JJ, et al. Diagnostic value of high signal abnormalities on T2 weighted MRI in the differentiation of Alzheimer's, frontotemporal, and vascular dementias. *Act Neurol Scand* 2002;105:355–364.
8. Erkinjuntti T, Kurz A, Gauthier S, et al. Efficacy of galantamine in probable vascular dementia and Alzheimer's disease combined with cerebrovascular disease: a randomized trial. *Lancet* 2002;359:1283–1290.
9. McKeith IG, Del Ser T, Spano P, et al. Efficacy of rivastigmine in dementia with Lewy bodies: a randomised, double-blind, placebo-controlled international study. *Lancet* 2000;356:2031–2036.
10. Rogers SL, Farlow MR, Doody RS, et al. Donepezil study group. A 24-week, double-blind, placebo-controlled trial of donepezil in patients with Alzheimer's disease. *Neurology* 1998;50:136–145.
11. Rosler M, Anand R, Veach J, et al. Efficacy and safety of rivastigmine in patients with Alzheimer's disease: international randomized controlled trial. *BMJ* 1999; 318:633–638.
12. Raskind MA, Peskind ER, Wessel T, et al. Galantamine in AD: a 6-month randomized, placebo-controlled trial with a 6-month extension. *Neurology* 2000;54:2261–2268.
13. Sano M, Ernesto C, Thomas RG, et al. A controlled trial of selegiline, alpha-tocopherol, or both as treatment for Alzheimer's disease. *N Engl J Med* 1997;336:1216–1222.

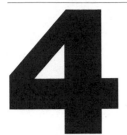

Delirium

Kyle C. Moylan

INTRODUCTION

Delirium is a common, frequently unrecognized, medical syndrome affecting up to 30% of hospitalized inpatients, with the elderly being at greatest risk. It may be the admitting diagnosis or a complication of a hospitalization for another condition. The DSM-IV lists formal criteria for the diagnosis of delirium (Table 4-1) or **acute confusional state**. It is important to identify and treat patients appropriately, as these patients are at risk for complications of their hospitalization such as dehydration, malnutrition, aspiration, skin ulcers, deconditioning, falls, institutionalization, and longer hospitalization. The mortality rate is also high (approximately 8%), which is in part related to the severity of the underlying medical conditions.

CLINICAL SUBTYPES

Delirium can be divided into hyperactive and hypoactive subtypes, based on the type of observed psychomotor activity. These can coexist in a single individual.

Hyperactive Delirium

Hyperactive delirium is the **most commonly recognized form** of delirium. Patients demonstrate agitation, psychosis, mood lability, refusal to cooperate with medical care, and other disruptive behaviors. Frequently, the house officer will be called to deal with a patient pulling out IVs and other catheters or trying to climb out of bed. Patients with delirium from anticholinergic agents, intoxications, and alcohol withdrawal usually present in this manner.

Hypoactive Delirium

Hypoactive delirium is the **most common form** of delirium but is less frequently recognized by clinicians. The patients are confused, lethargic, and sluggish. It may be mistaken for fatigue or somnolence but differs because the patient cannot be easily aroused and maintained in a normal level of consciousness with mild stimuli. Stronger stimuli are required for arousal, which is usually incomplete and transient. The underlying etiology for this pattern is often due to metabolic and other encephalopathies.

CAUSES

Pathophysiology

The pathophysiology of delirium has not been fully elucidated. It is thought to be due to a **generalized** disorder of cerebral metabolism and neurotransmission (bihemispheric dysfunction); however, **specific** neural pathways also seem to be important. This is evident because some medications with actions on specific pathways and neurotransmitters (i.e., anticholinergic drugs) are capable of precipitating delirium.

Differential Diagnosis

Delirium must be distinguished from other forms of global cognitive impairment.

TABLE 4-1. DSM-IV CRITERIA FOR DELIRIUM

Disturbance of consciousness
  Decreased level of awareness
  Impaired ability to focus attention
  Impaired ability to shift attention
Disturbance of cognition
  Memory deficits
  Disorientation
  Language disturbances
Develops over a short time period
  Hours to days
  Fluctuates over the course of the day; "sundowning"
Evidence that the above changes are a consequence of a general medical condition, intoxication, and/or medication

Dementia
Dementia (see Chap. 3, Dementia) differs because of its gradual onset (usually years) and persistence. **Dementia does not cause impaired alertness until the late stages** (should be obvious from collateral history). Patients with dementia are prone to delirium, however, and an acute worsening in a demented patient suggests delirium or another acute insult. **Dementia with Lewy bodies may present with hallucinations and psychosis early in its course.**

Depression
Depression (see Chap. 5, Depression in the Older Adult) **may mimic hypoactive delirium** with prominent withdrawal, psychomotor retardation, slowed speech, apathy, and pseudodementia. **Depression should not affect the level of consciousness.** A more prolonged course and a history of major depression may be helpful clues.

Psychosis
Psychosis **may mimic hyperactive delirium.** Functional psychosis is distinguishable by auditory hallucinations, more systematic delusions, and a less fluctuating course (less fluctuation throughout the course of a day).

Cerebrovascular Accident
Cerebrovascular accident (CVA) may rarely present with delirium or be mistaken for delirium. For example, receptive or expressive aphasia may be mistaken for confusion. Also, a diffuse attention disorder can result from a stroke in the temporooccipital, parietal, prefrontal, or subcortical regions of the right hemisphere. An acute illness may worsen the focal neurologic signs associated with old cerebrovascular events.

PRESENTATION
Clinical Characteristics

Impaired level of consciousness is a diagnostic characteristic. Patients have impaired alertness and difficulty concentrating. Ability to maintain and focus attention appropriately is affected, making patients easily distracted and unable to ignore irrelevant stimuli.

  Impaired cognition is also a key diagnostic feature. It is manifested by memory impairment (in part owing to problems with registering and processing information)

and disturbances in executive function. Patients have difficulty planning tasks and solving problems.
Perceptual disturbances and sensory features are common, especially in younger patients. They can be present in hyperactive and hypoactive forms. Hallucinations are most frequently visual (contrasted with the auditory hallucinations more common with schizophrenia). Paranoid and persecutory delusions may be present.
Somatic features predominate in older patients. These include urinary incontinence, gait impairments, tremor, language disorders (receptive or expressive aphasia), and sleep disorders (reversal of sleep patterns, brief and fragmented sleep). **Focal neurologic signs may be present but suggest an underlying CNS disorder.** Focal signs associated with a prior CVA will be exacerbated by an acute illness.
Emotional disturbances, such as mood lability and depression, may be present.

Risk Factors

Risk factors for the development of delirium include advanced age and dementia. In addition, each of the etiologies listed later can be thought of as a risk factor (Table 4-2).

EVALUATION

History

By the very nature of the problem, history taking is problematic in delirious patients. Patients are generally confused and poor historians; they will likely not recognize that a problem exists. Therefore, **collateral history is imperative.** History should be elicited from family members or other caregivers and should focus on several items (Table 4-3).

Physical Exam

The purpose of the physical exam in delirious patients is to **identify possible precipitating causes or evidence of a focal neurologic process.** The Confusion Assessment Method (CAM) is provided as a tool in Appendix D to aid in the assessment of the delirious patient.

TABLE 4-2. UNDERLYING ETIOLOGIES OF DELIRIUM

Infections: UTI, pneumonia

Medications: anticholinergics (antihistamines, clonidine, tricyclic antidepressants), narcotics (meperidine), benzodiazepines, H_2-blockers, steroids, theophylline, digoxin, antiparkinsonian agents, neuroleptic malignant syndrome

Withdrawal: ethanol, narcotics, benzodiazepines

Electrolyte abnormalities: especially hyper- or hyponatremia and hypercalcemia, but also consider overly rapid correction of hyper- or hypotonicity resulting in cerebral edema or central pontine myelinolysis

Postop: analgesics, hypotension, anesthesia, fluid and electrolyte abnormalities

Metabolic derangement: uremia, portosystemic encephalopathy, vitamin B_{12} deficiency, Wernicke-Korsakoff syndrome, hyper- or hypoglycemia, hyper- or hypothyroidism, hypoxia, hypercapnea

CNS disorders: cerebrovascular accident, vasculitis, subdural hematoma, neoplasia (primary or metastatic), meningitis, encephalitis, neurosyphilis, relative hypotension

Environmental: hyperthermia, hypothermia, trauma, burns, fractures

TABLE 4-3. KEY HISTORICAL FEATURES

Baseline mental status (Has there been evidence of progressive cognitive decline suggesting dementia?)
Previous history of delirium
History of falls or head injury
Medications (prescription and over-the-counter), especially recent changes
Ethanol use

Vital signs may point to a specific underlying problem. On complete physical exam, look for evidence of infections, dehydration, and head trauma. Evaluate for fecal impaction or urinary retention.

The **Short Blessed Test** (see Appendix A) can be a useful screen for cognitive dysfunction and has the advantage of being widely known, making communication between physicians easier A score of >8 is abnormal, but false-negatives can occur. A single normal exam does not exclude the diagnosis, as it does not take into account fluctuations in mental status, or abnormalities in speech, behavior, or motor activity. Also, the Short Blessed Test does not distinguish acute from chronic processes. Serial exams are likely to be more useful to identify delirious patients and follow their clinical course, and, for this reason, **a baseline Short Blessed Test on admission for all patients with the diagnosis of delirium or at high risk for developing delirium is useful.**

Passive exam of patient behaviors is important to observe and document:

- **Motor activity:** Is there excess activity such as fidgeting or pulling at IVs or clothing (psychomotor agitation), or is there lack of activity (psychomotor retardation)?
- **Alertness:** Is the patient lethargic? What level of stimuli is required to arouse the patient, and how long does it last?
- **Attentiveness:** Can the patient maintain focus during a conversation, or is he or she easily distracted by the surroundings? Can the patient shift attention appropriately to new stimuli?
- **Speech:** Pay attention to content. Is the patient suspicious or delusional?
  - Pay attention to the flow of thought. Is the patient tangential or perseverating?
  - Is there slurring of the speech to indicate an acute or old cerebrovascular event?

Etiology

Once a diagnosis of delirium has been established, the focus should shift to identifying and **treating the underlying cause,** while supporting the patient and providing a safe environment. Common causes of delirium include UTIs, pneumonia, fecal impaction, hypoxia, relative hypotension, medications (especially anticholinergics), and withdrawal (Table 4-3), but there may be multiple underlying etiologies.

Diagnostic Workup

Basic Lab Studies

Basic labs include UA with microscopic analysis (culture if abnormal), electrolytes (including calcium and BUN/Cr), liver panel, and CBC. A chest radiograph should be a routine part of the evaluation to exclude unsuspected pneumonia. Consider further testing, when appropriate, with arterial blood gases, ECG, ethanol level, and toxicology screens.

Neuroimaging Studies

A noncontrast head CT should be performed if there are new focal neurologic deficits (to evaluate for old cerebrovascular disease, acute intracranial hemorrhage, or other structural abnormality) or if there is a history of falls (to exclude a subdural hematoma). MRI may be indicated to evaluate for an acute CVA in patients with suggestive clinical findings.

Lumbar Puncture

Lumbar puncture to exclude meningoencephalitis is indicated for patients with unexplained mental status changes, especially in the face of fever, leukocytosis, or other evidence of sepsis that is not readily attributable to another source of infection. Failure to perform a lumbar puncture in the appropriate setting may not only lead to delays in effective antimicrobial treatment with increased mortality but will also contribute to diagnostic and therapeutic uncertainties if the patient does not respond as expected to empiric therapies.

Electroencephalogram

EEG is not routinely indicated but can be useful in cases in which the diagnosis remains in doubt, or there is concern for seizure activity. The findings of delirium are typically nonspecific, diffuse slow-wave activity.

MANAGEMENT

Treatment

- **Treatment is primarily supportive until the underlying precipitants are identified and treated.**
- Review medications; give a therapeutic and diagnostic trial of stopping suspect medications. Avoid starting new medications that could worsen the problem.
- Use specialized geriatric care units (i.e., acute care for the elderly unit, see Chap. 2, Settings for Geriatric Care) when available.
- Maximize the safety of the surrounding environment: "fall precautions."
- **Avoid physical restraints,** which can result in iatrogenic injuries.
- Avoid interrupting sleep (order a time period at night uninterrupted by vital signs).
- Increase activity and mobility in the daytime.
- Provide sitters (especially familiar faces—ask family members to stay with the patient).
- Evaluate sensory input:
  - Avoid sensory extremes.
  - Avoid placing two delirious patients in the same room.
  - Provide hearing and visual aids (have family bring from home if necessary).
  - Use windows to orient patient to the day/night cycle.
  - Is the patient in pain?
- Document the diagnosis and the clinical findings in the chart to assist cross-covering physicians. When signing out the patient, note patients at risk for delirium and specific interventions to be undertaken.

Pharmacologic Interventions

Not every patient with delirium requires specific pharmacologic treatment. Medications are indicated for specific disruptive or harmful behaviors but do not alter the course of delirium. Medications should only be given in conjunction with nonpharmacologic measures (Table 4-4).

Neuroleptic agents may be useful in treating hyperactive patients who represent a danger to themselves or the staff. They have little effect on respiratory drive and BP. Avoid their use in patients with parkinsonism. Possible adverse reactions include dystonias, akathisia (can mimic delirium), catatonia, tardive dyskinesia, and neuroleptic malignant syndrome. **Haloperidol (Haldol) is the drug of choice for treatment of hyperactive delirium.** Initially administered IM/IV for prompt control, the starting dose should be low (0.5–1 mg) given parenterally, which can be doubled qh until control is achieved. Depending on the patient's course, repeated doses can then be given q4–8h and then switched to PO administration if continued maintenance is needed. For conversion, give 50–100% of the parenteral dose required in 24 hrs divided up bid or tid. Newer, atypical antipsychotics do not appear to be any more effective.

Intermediate-acting benzodiazepines can be useful adjuncts to antipsychotic agents. They are particularly indicated for severe agitation, insomnia, and withdrawal syndromes. Benzodiazepines may have a more rapid onset of action than antipsychotics when

TABLE 4-4. PHARMACOLOGIC INTERVENTIONS IN PATIENTS WITH DELIRIUM

	Half-life (hrs)	Elimination	Dosing	Contraindications	Adverse Effects	Interactions
Neuroleptics						
Haloperidol (Haldol)	18	Hepatic	IM/IV[a]—0.5–10 mg as often as qh until response, then q4–8h[b] PO—equivalent dose divided bid or tid	QT prolongation, parkinsonism	Tardive dyskinesia, akithisia, dystonia, neuroleptic malignant syndrome, QT prolongation, dry mouth, urinary retention, possible aspiration	Potentiates other CNS depressants
Benzodiazepines						
Lorazepam (Ativan)	14	Hepatic with renal elimination of inactive metabolite	IM/IV—0.5–2 mg up to tid PO—0.5–2 mg up to tid	Sleep apnea, respiratory insufficiency	Confusion, delirium, lethargy, ataxia	Potentiates other CNS depressants; valproate increases lorazepam levels

[a]IV not FDA approved.
[b]Up to 100 mg in 24 hrs.

administered parenterally but cause more sedation and respiratory depression. **Some patients with delirium may have a paradoxic increase in agitation when given benzodiazepines.** Intermediate-acting agents are preferable [lorazepam (Ativan)], as short-acting agents risk causing a paradoxical agitation after drug withdrawal. Initial dose in the geriatric patient should be 0.5–2 mg of lorazepam (parenteral or PO). Adverse reactions include respiratory depression, hypotension, and delirium. **Pain control in a delirious patient is a difficult management issue.** Although pain may be a cause of delirium, opioid analgesics may exacerbate the problem. A reasonable approach is to treat the patients' pain with nonnarcotic agents initially; if unsuccessful, follow with a trial of a short-acting agent such as fentanyl and follow the clinical response closely.

Natural Course and Follow-Up

The natural course of delirium is widely variable and partially dependent on the underlying etiology. The course tends to fluctuate over hours and days; the severity and manifestations are vastly different at different times. Although the course should improve with treatment of the triggering cause, **signs and symptoms may persist for weeks and even months after the initial event.** Many patients have underlying dementia, but the initial diagnosis should generally be deferred 3–6 mos after an episode of delirium to allow full recovery.

KEY POINTS TO REMEMBER

* Delirium is a common and serious condition in the elderly with a high mortality rate.
* Delirium is characterized by disturbances of cognition and consciousness, a fluctuating course, and one or multiple precipitants.
* Delirium can be hyperactive or hypoactive. Hypoactive delirium is more frequently unrecognized.
* The primary treatment of delirium is supportive care while the underlying cause is sought and treated.
* Always review the patient's medications for possible contributors to delirium. Be particularly alert to recent medication changes.
* Physical restraints frequently result in iatrogenic injuries and should be avoided.
* Pharmacologic intervention with neuroleptics or benzodiazepines should be reserved for short-term use to treat specific disruptive or harmful behaviors.

REFERENCES AND SUGGESTED READINGS

Espino DV, Jules-Bradley AC, Johnston CL, et al. Diagnostic approach to the confused elderly patient. *Am Fam Phys* 1998:57:1358–1366.
Inouye SK, Bogardus ST Jr, Charpentier PA, et al. A multicomponent intervention to prevent delirium in hospitalized older patient. *N Engl J Med* 1999;340;669–676.
Meagher D. Delirium: optimising management. *BMJ* 2001;322:144–149.
Rummans T, Evans JM, Krahn LE, et al. Delirium in elderly patients: evaluation and management. *Mayo Clin Proc* 1995;70:989–998.
Tune L. Delirium. In: Hazzard WR, Ouslander JG, Blass JP, et al., eds. *Principles of geriatric medicine and gerontology*, 4th ed. New York: McGraw-Hill, 1999:1229–1237.

Depression in the Older Adult

Kyle C. Moylan

INTRODUCTION

Depression affects 10–15% of the outpatient geriatric population and >20% of the geriatric inpatients. **Depression is not a result of normal aging;** untreated depression leads to functional decline, cognitive impairment, social isolation, and an increased risk of morbidity and mortality from coexisting illnesses. Depression is a risk factor for subsequent Alzheimer's disease and cerebrovascular disease. **Many cases go unrecognized,** in part because patients may have atypical presentations compared to their younger counterparts. Identification of depression is vital, because treatment is effective for most patients.

PRESENTATION

Clinical Features

Table 5-1 **lists the classic neurovegetative symptoms of major depression.** In the geriatric population, patients may have symptoms such as anxiety, somatic complaints, or frank psychosis (especially delusions). **Elderly patients are more likely to present with weight loss** (see Chap. 9, Unintentional Weight Loss in the Elderly).

Depression and dementia frequently coexist in the same patient (see Chap. 3, Dementia). Depression is common in patients with dementia, who may present atypically by wandering, by crying out, with aggression, or with functional decline. The diagnosis can be difficult, because some neurovegetative symptoms may develop in uncomplicated dementia. **Depression itself can cause cognitive impairment (pseudodementia) that may be reversible.** Differentiating between the two scenarios can be difficult, and there is no way to accurately predict which patients treated with antidepressants will show cognitive improvement. Pseudodemented patients are more likely to complain of cognitive difficulties than are patients with true dementia.

Many patients do not meet criteria for major depression but exhibit disabling subsyndromal symptoms of depression. **Patients with multiple symptoms who do not meet criteria for major depression** have comparable outcomes to those who do and therefore **should be treated.**

Risk Factors

Age alone does not appear to be a risk factor for depression in community-dwelling elderly. Nursing home residents and hospitalized patients are at increased risk, as are those with **multiple medical problems.** Other risk factors include a history of depression, a family history of depression, Parkinson's disease, and stroke.

EVALUATION

Diagnosis and Screening

The most important step in managing depression is identifying affected patients. It is particularly important to consider the diagnosis in several clinical situations (Table 5-2). Any comprehensive geriatric assessment usually includes a screening test for depression. **It is feasible to quickly screen all geriatric patients for depression, because two simple**

TABLE 5-1. DEPRESSIVE SYMPTOMS[a]

Symptom	Features
Depressed mood	Depressed mood most of the day, nearly every day
Anhedonia	Markedly diminished interest or pleasure in almost all activities
Weight change	Substantial unintentional weight loss or gain
Sleep disturbance	Insomnia or hypersomnia nearly every day
Psychomotor problems	Psychomotor agitation or retardation nearly every day
Lack of energy	Fatigue or loss of energy nearly every day
Excessive guilt	Feelings of worthlessness or excessive guilt nearly every day
Poor concentration	Diminished ability to think or concentrate nearly every day
Suicidal ideation	Recurrent thoughts about death or suicide

[a]DSM-IV diagnostic criteria for major depression requires five or more depressive symptoms, including depressed mood or anhedonia, lasting ≥ 2 wks.
From *Diagnostic and statistical manual of mental disorders*, 4th ed. Text revision. Washington, DC: American Psychiatric Association, 1994, with permission.

questions will identify up to 95% of patients with major depression in the outpatient setting:

• During the past month, have you often been bothered by feeling down, depressed, or hopeless?
• During the past month, have you often been bothered by having little interest or pleasure in doing things?

If the answer to both questions is no, depression is very unlikely. If the answer to either question is yes, a more thorough evaluation is indicated.

Suicide

Specifically inquire about suicidal ideation. Elderly patients are at a higher risk for committing suicide, with elderly white men living alone being at the greatest risk. Risk factors include male gender, white race, social isolation, previous suicide attempts or inpatient psychiatric care, substance abuse, a specific plan for committing suicide, and access to firearms. Most patients who attempt suicide seek help from their primary care providers in the previous month, and many are coping with their first episode of depression.

History

The history should elicit the nature of the symptoms mentioned earlier, medications, past suicide attempts, psychiatric history, and the use of alcohol or drugs. It

TABLE 5-2. INDICATIONS TO SCREEN FOR DEPRESSION

Cognitive dysfunction	Weight loss
Multiple medical problems	Functional decline
Chronic pain	Frequent hospitalizations
Personal or family history of depression	Parkinson's disease
Unexplained physical symptoms	Stroke
Anxiety disorders	

is important to identify patients with coexisting mania or psychosis, as the management is different. Collateral history is important in patients with cognitive dysfunction. Inventory tools, such as the **Geriatric Depression Scale** (see Appendix C), are available to further evaluate the likelihood of depression and document symptoms that can be followed over time. Keep in mind that dementia may impair the patient's ability to answer screening questions appropriately, reinforcing the importance of collateral history.

Physical Exam and Lab Evaluation

Physical exam should focus on signs of systemic illnesses, as well as on assessment of cognitive function and fall risk. **The only lab test that is routinely part of the evaluation is TSH, but a more complete battery may identify a previously unrecognized condition that is contributing (CBC, electrolytes, calcium, liver function, vitamin B$_{12}$, 25-OH vitamin D, testosterone, and UA).** There is no indication for neuroimaging, but depressed elderly patients are more likely to have abnormal studies with nonspecific findings.

MANAGEMENT

Treatment

The treatment of depressed geriatric patients should be part of a comprehensive plan of care. In some situations, such as bereavement or depression of short duration, watchful waiting may be the best approach. The potential risks and benefits of different treatments must be considered so that treatment can be tailored to the individual patient. Initial therapy with antidepressants or structured psychotherapy can be effective in at least one-half of patients, and the combination may be most effective. **Compliance with psychotherapy and medications is problematic, so discussing the patient's preference is essential.** Indications to refer to a psychiatrist are listed in Table 5-3.

Nonpharmacologic treatment is important. A key principle is to educate the family and caregivers about the role of depression in the current clinical context, what the available treatment options are (including expected time to achieve results and possible side effects), and what the expected benefits will be. Structured psychotherapy is an effective option for patients with adequate cognitive function and is probably underused because of the widespread availability of antidepressants.

Pharmacotherapy

The elderly respond to pharmacologic treatment as well as younger patients. No single drug has been shown to be any more effective than another for depressive symptoms, so **the choice of antidepressant (Table 5-4) should be based on the side effect profile, drug interactions, response to previous treatments, and associated conditions** (anxiety disorder, obsessive-compulsive disorder, chronic pain). In general, tricyclic antidepressants are avoided in the elderly because of anticholinergic and antihistamine side effects,

TABLE 5-3. INDICATIONS FOR REFERRAL TO A PSYCHIATRIST

History of mania

Psychosis

Severe depression

Severe psychomotor retardation

Possible need for inpatient psychiatric care or electroconvulsive therapy

Suicidal ideation

Failure to respond to initial treatment

TABLE 5-4. CHARACTERISTIC OF VARIOUS ANTIDEPRESSANTS

Class	Drug	Initial dosage (PO)	Target dosage (PO)	Step-up dose (PO)	Other indications	Drug-specific side effects
TCA						
Tertiary amine	Amitriptyline (Elavil, Endep)	25 mg qhs	100 mg qhs	150 mg qhs	Chronic pain, insomnia	TCA class effects
Secondary amine	Nortriptyline (Aventyl, Pamelor)	25 mg qhs	50–75 mg qhs	100–150 mg qhs	ADD, IBS, neuropathic pain	TCA class effects
Serotonin and norepinephrine reuptake inhibitors	Venlafaxine (Effexor) (Effexor XR)	37.5 mg bid 37.5 mg qd	75 mg bid 75 mg qd	100–150 mg bid 225 mg qd	Anxiety disorder, neuropathic pain, OCD	Dose-dependent rise in DBP, nausea, somnolence, insomnia, sexual dysfunction
Selective serotonin reuptake inhibitor (SSRI)	Citalopram (Celexa)	10 mg qd	20 mg qd	40 mg qd	OCD, panic disorder	SSRI class effects, few drug interactions
	Escitalopram (Lexapro)	5 mg qd	10 mg qd	20 mg qd	—	L-Isomer of citalopram, SSRI class effects, few drug interactions
	Paroxetine (Paxil)	20 mg qd	20 mg qd	50 mg qd	OCD, panic disorder; social phobia, migraine	SSRI class effects
	Sertraline (Zoloft)	25–50 mg qd	100 mg qd	150–200 mg qd	OCD, PTSD, panic disorder	SSRI class effects
Serotonin antagonist	Mirtazapine (Remeron)	7.5–15 mg qhs	30 mg qhs	45 mg qhs	Anxiety, insomnia	Sedation, increased appetite, weight gain, dry mouth, dizziness

(continued)

TABLE 5-4. CONTINUED

Class	Drug	Initial dosage (PO)	Target dosage (PO)	Step-up dose (PO)	Other indications	Drug-specific side effects
Norepinephrine and dopamine reuptake inhibitors	Bupropion (Wellbutrin)	75 mg bid	150 mg bid	150 mg tid	Smoking cessation, PTSD, attention deficit disorder	Agitation, anxiety, insomnia, anorexia, constipation, tremor, seizures
	(Wellbutrin SR)	150 mg qam	150 mg bid	200 mg bid		
Serotonin antagonists and reuptake inhibitors	Trazodone (Desyrel)	50 mg qhs	200 mg qhs	200 mg bid	Insomnia	Priapism, drowsiness, headache, GI upset, orthostasis

OCD, obsessive-compulsive disorder; PTSD, posttraumatic stress disorder; TCA, tricyclic antidepressant.
Adapted from Whooley MA, Simon GE. Managing depression in medical outpatients. *N Engl J Med* 2000;343:1942–1950.

including orthostatic hypotension, delirium, and cognitive dysfunction. Of the SSRIs, fluoxetine (Prozac) is avoided in the elderly because of its long half-life, multiple drug interactions, and potential to exacerbate anorexia and weight loss (see Appendix E for common CYP450 interactions). Common side effects of SSRIs include sleep disturbances, weight gain or weight loss, falls, sweating, fatigue, diarrhea, and sexual dysfunction.

In elderly patients, the medication should be started at the lowest dose and titrated up to a target dose over the next 2 wks. Follow-up (by telephone or in person) should be provided after approximately 4 wks, because the onset of action is between 1 and 3 wks. If there is no improvement and side effects are tolerable, the dose can be increased to a step-up dose (above which there would be no further expected benefit). If there is still no response, consider switching to a different agent (although switching classes is not necessary). Patient contact should continue every few weeks until an improvement occurs. **Antidepressants may take 6 wks or longer to have a full therapeutic effect.**

Adjunctive therapy should be considered in those patients with inadequate response to antidepressants. Estrogen replacement, liothyronine (Cytomel), and vitamin D have been reported to enhance the response to antidepressants.

Methylphenidate (Ritalin) has been used as a stimulant for depressed patients with severe psychomotor retardation, although data supporting its use are limited. The initial dosage is 5 mg PO bid, which can be increased to 10 mg PO bid if there is no initial response. A response is usually evident within a few days. Contraindications include confusion, cardiovascular disease, and arrhythmias.

Electroconvulsive therapy is indicated for severe depression that fails medical treatment. It can also be used when a more immediate effect is needed or in patients with associated psychosis or catatonia. Memory loss and confusion can occur and usually resolve within a week. Contraindications include increased intracranial pressure, space-occupying brain lesions, and recent MI or stroke.

Treatment should continue for at least 6 mos to prevent relapse. For patients with recurrent depression, treatment should continue for at least 2 yrs, if not indefinitely. Discontinuation should occur by tapering the dose over 2–3 mos with frequent follow-up. Abrupt discontinuation of short-acting serotonergic drugs may result in a **serotonin syndrome** (tinnitus, vertigo, or paresthesias). Approximately one-third will have relapse of their depression in the first year after discontinuation, underscoring the fact that depression becomes a chronic illness for many patients.

Frequent mistakes in the management of depression include failure to reach a therapeutic antidepressant dose, inadequate dose titration, inadequate follow-up, and failure to educate the patient about the illness and treatment.

KEY POINTS TO REMEMBER

* Depression is very common in the geriatric population.
* Depression is frequently unrecognized or undertreated.
* Two simple questions will identify up to 95% of patients with major depression.
* Symptoms of depression may be atypical in the elderly, including cognitive impairment, anxiety, weight loss, psychosis, aggression, functional decline, or somatic complaints.
* Geriatric patients with depression are at high risk for suicide, cardiovascular disease, dementia, and disability.
* Antidepressants and psychotherapy are effective in the elderly. Other adjunctive therapies may also be appropriate.

WEB RESOURCES

American Medical Association (http://www.medem.com/MedLB/articleslb.cfm?sub_cat=128).
Depression Awareness, Recognition, and Treatment program of the National Institute of Mental Health (http://www.nimh.nih.gov/publicat/index.cfm).
National Depressive and Manic-Depressive Association (http://www.dbsalliance.org/).
National Foundation for Depressive Illness (http://www.depression.org/).

National Mental Health Association (http://www.nmha.org/ccd).

Psychology Information Online (http://www.psychologyinfo.com/depression).

SUGGESTED READING

Drugs for depression and anxiety. *Med Lett Drugs Ther* 1999;41:33–38.

Koenig HG. Late-life depression: how to treat patients with chronic illness. *Geriatrics* 1999;54:56–62.

Menza AM, Liberatore BL. Psychiatry in the geriatric neurology practice. *Neurol Clin North Am* 1998;16:611–634.

Shankar KK, Orrell MW. Detecting and managing depression and anxiety in people with dementia. *Curr Opin Psychiatry* 2000;13:55–59.

Sheikh JI, Yesavage JA. Geriatric depression scale: recent evidence and development of a shorter version. *Clin Gerontol* 1986;5:165–172.

Sutor B, Rummans TA, Jowsey SG, et al. Major depression in medically ill patients. *Mayo Clin Proc* 1998;73:329–337.

Whooley MA, Avins AL, et al. Case-finding instruments for depression: two questions are as good as many. *J Gen Intern Med* 1997;12:439–445.

Whooley MA, Simon GE. Managing depression in medical outpatients. *N Engl J Med* 2000;343:1942–1950.

REFERENCE

1. Whooley MA, Avins AL, Miranda J, et al. Case-finding instruments for depression: two questions are as good as many. *J Gen Intern Med* 1997;12:439–445.

Approach to Polypharmacy and Appropriate Medication Use

Randall Wooley and
Kyle C. Moylan

INTRODUCTION

Optimal use of medications in the elderly can be difficult and requires attention to the changes in body composition and physiology that accompany aging. It is complicated by the fact that most elderly patients are on several medications at any given time. In the United States, **patients >65 yrs fill an average of 12 prescriptions per year** compared with five by those aged 25–44 yrs. As more drugs become available and longevity continues to increase, it can be expected that the incidence of polypharmacy and inappropriate medication use will grow.

Use of nonprescription medications is more common in the elderly. Adverse drug reactions may also be more common in the elderly, whereas **drug-drug interactions** are definitely more common. The increased frequency of adverse drug reactions is a reflection of comorbidities and polypharmacy as well as age-related changes. The elderly population is very heterogeneous, which means that efficacy and toxicity of the same medication will vary widely from patient to patient. **Polypharmacy** increases the risk of cognitive impairment and falls. **Adherence** to a prescribed regimen can often be difficult because of cognitive deficits, visual problems, financial difficulties, and complicated regimens.

PHARMACOKINETICS AND AGING

Age-related and pathologic changes in physiology and body composition occur in the elderly. These alterations affect absorption, distribution, metabolism, and excretion of individual drugs. (See Appendix E for specific formulas)

Absorption is affected by changes in gastric pH. For example, **achlorhydria is more common in the elderly** (occurring in 20–25% of individuals >80 yrs), decreasing the serum levels of drugs that are dependent on gastric pH for absorption (e.g., ketoconazole, fluconazole, tetracycline). Decreased splanchnic blood flow and GI motility may also decrease absorption, but these changes for the most part are not thought to be clinically significant.

There is an age-related decline in lean body mass and subsequent increase in body fat (in older men, the percentage of body mass that is fat can increase to $\geq 33\%$, and for women, 40–50%). Total body water also decreases with age. **These changes result in a decreased volume of distribution (Vd) for hydrophilic drugs and an increase in Vd for lipophilic drugs.** This means that lipophilic benzodiazepines will have a longer half life in older adults due to an increased Vd. On the other hand, the Vd for hydrophilic drugs, such as ethanol and digoxin, is decreased and results in a higher level given the same amount of drug. In addition, **serum albumin levels tend to decrease with age,** leading to higher free levels of highly protein-bound drugs (e.g., digoxin, theophylline, warfarin, and phenytoin).

Alterations in metabolism occur as a result of decreased hepatic mass and blood flow. Drugs with a first-pass effect in the liver may be effective at lower doses (e.g., beta blockers, nitrates, calcium channel blockers, and tricyclic antidepressants). Cytochrome P450 oxidation declines with aging, and drug-drug interactions involving these enzymes are important to recognize (see Appendix E).

Excretion is altered as a result of the change in renal structure and function. Several structural and functional changes accompany the aging process. These include a loss of renal mass, obliteration of afferent arterioles in the cortex, increased number of sclerosed glomeruli, reduction in the number of tubules, interstitial fibrosis, and a decline in renal blood flow and glomerular filtration rate (GFR). **A decrease in GFR of approximately 10 mL/min/decade after the fourth decade of life has been observed.** An increase in serum creatinine may not be noted, because there is a proportional decrease in lean body mass. Keep these changes in mind when prescribing medications that are renally cleared (e.g., aminoglycosides, acyclovir, amantadine, digoxin, lithium, atenolol, and vancomycin).

PHARMACODYNAMICS AND AGING

Aging is also associated with changes in the end-organ responsiveness to drugs at the receptor or postreceptor level. For example, there is decreased sensitivity to beta receptors with aging along with a possible decreased clinical response to beta blockers and beta-agonists. Increased sensitivity to drugs such as opiates and warfarin has also been noted.

ADVERSE DRUG REACTIONS

Adverse drug reactions represent the most common form of iatrogenic illness. One-fourth of hospitalized patients >80 yrs experience an adverse drug reaction compared to one-tenth of those aged 40–50. **Risk factors for adverse drug reactions** include age, polypharmacy, female gender, lower body weight, hepatic or renal insufficiency, and history of drug reactions. Many medications are frequently implicated in adverse reactions and should be avoided in the elderly (Table 6-1).

TABLE 6-1. KEY DRUGS TO AVOID IN THE ELDERLY

Benzodiazepines	**Antihistamines**
Diazepam (Valium)	Diphenhydramine (Benadryl)
Chlordiazepoxide (Librium)	Chlorpheniramine (Chlor-Trimeton)
Alprazolam (Xanax)	Cimetidine (Tagamet)
Flurazepam (Dalmane)	**Antidepressants**
Barbiturates	Amitriptyline (Elavil) and other tricyclics
Pentobarbital (Nembutal)	Combination antidepressant/antipsychotics
Secobarbital (Seconal)	**Antispasmodics (anticholinergic)**
Analgesics	Belladonna (Donnatal)
Meperidine (Demerol)	Dicyclomine (Bentyl)
Propoxyphene (Darvocet)	Hyoscyamine (Levsin)
NSAIDs	Clidinium (Librax)
Muscle relaxants	Oxybutynin (Ditropan)
Cyclobenzaprine (Flexeril)	Tolterodine (Detrol)
Methocarbamol	**Cardiovascular**
Carisoprodol	Methyldopa (Aldomet)
Antiemetics/prokinetics	Reserpine (Serpasil)
Trimethobenzamide (Tigan)	Propanolol
Promethazine (Phenergan)	Digoxin (especially >0.125 mg qd)
Metoclopramide (Reglan)	Dipyridamole

TABLE 6-2. COMMON DRUG-DISEASE INTERACTIONS TO AVOID

Disease	Drugs to avoid
Congestive heart failure	Disopyramide, drugs with high sodium content, NSAIDs, calcium channel blockers
Diabetes mellitus	Beta blockers if hypoglycemia is a problem, corticosteroids
COPD	Beta blockers, sedative-hypnotics, opiates
Asthma	Beta blockers
Ulcers	NSAIDs, ASA, potassium, corticosteroids
Seizures	Neuroleptics
Clotting disorder	ASA, NSAIDs, vitamin E, ticlopidine, warfarin
BPH	Anticholinergics, antihistamines, GI antispasmodic drugs, muscle relaxants, oxybutynin, narcotics, bethanechol
Incontinence	Alpha blockers
Constipation	See BPH; also calcium channel blockers, iron
Arrhythmias	TCAs, typical neuroleptics
Insomnia	Decongestants, theophylline, SSRI, beta-agonists
Cognitive dysfunction	Anticholinergics, antihistamines, TCAs, antispasmodics
Osteoporosis	Corticosteroids, anticonvulsants (see Chap. 14, Osteoporosis)

BPH, benign prostatic hyperplasia; TCAs, tricyclic antidepressants.

GUIDELINES FOR OPTIMAL PHARMACOTHERAPY

For the first patient encounter and each subsequent visit, a comprehensive review of medication use is warranted.

Identify all of the medications the patient is taking (prescription and nonprescription). The medications should be reviewed on a regular basis. It is advisable to have the patient or caretaker bring all medications to the office with them on every visit. If it is still unclear what the patient is actually taking, contacting the patient's pharmacy and family can provide useful information.

Communicate with other prescribers and consultants. **Communicate** with the patient and caregivers.

Keep a list of active medications readily available in the chart to review every visit. It may be helpful to list the indication for every prescription to ensure that there are no unnecessary medications.

Use **nonpharmacologic approaches** to treatment when available. ✓

Minimize the number of pills taken. Choose once-daily formulations when available. Maximize the dosage of one medication before adding second agents for the same purpose.

Encourage the use of a pillbox or other system to avoid confusion. Use home health services when available.

Avoid medications with common adverse effects in the elderly (i.e., falls, incontinence, and cognitive dysfunction, Table 6-1).

Keep a **current estimation of renal function** (calculated or measured GFR) available when prescribing renally cleared or potentially nephrotoxic medications.

Inquire about adverse effects from prescriptions regularly. Consider adverse effects in the differential diagnosis of any new symptom. Do not treat adverse effects from one medication with a second medication.

Identify financial barriers to compliance (including transportation to the pharmacy). Web sites listed later may be helpful for identifying prescription assistance programs.

When prescribing a new medication, review all of the available options, past adverse reactions, and potential drug-drug interactions (see Appendix E). Also consider drug-illness interactions (Table 6-2) and establish measurable end points for drug efficacy or failure.

Avoid generic drugs when there is a narrow therapeutic index. Examples include warfarin, digoxin, thyroxine, anticonvulsants, and antiarrhythmic agents.

Geriatricians must frequently reconcile established or possible efficacy of a drug with the patient's unique situation and goals.

KEY POINTS TO REMEMBER

* Polypharmacy is an important phenomenon in the elderly and contributes to adverse drug reactions.
* The elderly are a heterogeneous population with variable alterations in pharmacokinetics and pharmacodynamics.
* Consider adverse drug reactions whenever a new symptom develops in the geriatric patient.
* Avoid drugs that commonly cause adverse reactions in the elderly.
* Review medication use at every visit. Document the regimen, including over-the-counter medication. Specifically ask about adverse reactions and compliance.
* Facilitate patient compliance and adherence: communicate clearly, keep regimens simple, use the help of caregivers and home health, keep patient costs down, and use a pillbox or calendar.
* When starting a new drug, start at the lowest effective dose and titrate up slowly.

WEB RESOURCES

For Patients: Prescription Assistance

http://www.rxassist.org
http://www.rxhope.com
http://www.needymeds.com

For Health Care Professionals: Drug Interactions

http://www.drugfacts.com, http://www.handango.com, http://www.e-medtools.com
http://www.Rxcrosscheck.com ($20 fee)
http://www.medscape.com
http://www.fda.gov/cder/drug/mederrors
http://www.skyscape.com for PDA drug interaction programs and also http://www.epocrates.com

REFERENCES AND SUGGESTED READINGS

Avorn J, Gurwitx JH. Drug use in the nursing home. *Ann Intern Med* 1995;123:195–204.
Beck LH. The aging kidney: defending a delicate balance of fluid and electrolytes. *Geriatrics* 2000;55:26–33.
Beers MH. Explicit criteria for determining potentially inappropriate medication use by the elderly. *Arch Intern Med* 1907;157:1531–1536.
Chutka DS, Evans JM, Fleming KC, et al. Drug prescribing for elderly patients. *Mayo Clin Proc* 1995;70:685–693.
Evans JG, Williams TF, Beattie BL, et al. *Oxford textbook of geriatric medicine*, 2nd ed. New York: Oxford University Press, 2000.
Pannu N, Holloran PF. The kidney in aging. In: Greenberg A, ed. *Primer on kidney diseases*, 3rd ed. San Diego: Academic Press, 2001.

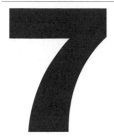

Falls

Monique Williams

INTRODUCTION

A fall is defined as an unintentional positional change that results in a person coming to rest on the ground, floor, or other lower level. Falls are one of the most common and serious problems affecting the elderly. Among community-dwelling persons >65 yrs, 30–60% fall annually, and one-half of these individuals fall more than once. Usually, multiple risk factors interact to precipitate falls. **Most falls occur in the home** (most often in the kitchen or bathroom) and typically occur while involved in normal activities of daily living. **Falls are a marker for poor health and functional decline and may be the presenting symptom of an acute or new illness.**

CONSEQUENCES OF FALLING

Falls have a significant impact on the health care system as well as the individual. **Accidents are the fifth leading cause of death in the elderly,** and fall-related injuries currently account for 6% of all medical expenditures.

The falling elderly face increased risk of hospitalization, nursing home admission, and death with each fall. One-third of long-term care facility admissions are related to falls in previously independent individuals.

Fear of falling can lead not only to recurrent falls but also decreased independence and self-imposed restriction of activities. Among elderly who fall, 10–25% limit their activity and consequently may precipitate functional decline.

5% of falls lead to fracture, with hip fracture accounting for 1% of complications. 5–10% of falls cause restricted activity for several days because of significant nonfracture injuries such as hematoma or sprain. The more severe fall complications include subdural hematoma and cervical fracture.

ETIOLOGIES AND RISK FACTORS FOR FALLS

The risk of falling increases with age. Proper gait and balance depend on correct integrated function of sensory, central, and musculoskeletal components. Aging and disease impair function of these components.

Aging impacts fall risk because of impaired postural reflexes, increased central processing time, decreased step length, decreased gait velocity, and decreased muscle mass.

Sensory changes that may be involved include impaired vestibular function, tactile sensation, proprioception, visual acuity, and dark adaptation.

There is a higher prevalence of **musculoskeletal disorders** in the elderly that can lead to joint stiffness and pain.

Risk factors for falls can be categorized as intrinsic, extrinsic, and environmental (Table 7-1). **Falls are typically multifactorial** and reflect the effect of multiple factors in addition to the age-related changes mentioned earlier. Single causes of falls include stroke, cerebellar dysfunction, parkinsonian disorders (see Chap. 26, Parkinson's Disease and Related Disorders), normal pressure hydrocephalus, and myelopathy. **Many of these risk factors can be modified, and it is the role of the clinician to**

TABLE 7-1.   RISK FACTORS FOR FALLS

Intrinsic risk factors	Hemiplegia and stroke
Older age	Peripheral neuropathy or myelopathy
Female gender	Fear of falling[a]
Vitamin D deficiency	Parkinsonism[a]
Lower extremity weakness[a]	**Extrinsic risk factors**
Poor grip strength[a]	Polypharmacy (≥ 4 medications)[a]
Balance disorder[a]	Specific drug classes[a]
Cognitive impairment[a]	Intoxication or withdrawal[a]
Podiatric problems[a]	Hospitalization or institutionalization
Visual deficits[a]	Recent hospitalization
Low gait speed	**Environmental risk factors**
Low body mass index[a]	Poor lighting[a]
Incontinence[a]	Loose carpets[a]
Depression[a]	Lack of bathroom safety equipment[a]
Hypotension, including postural[a]	

[a]Indicates risk factors that may be modifiable.

address and modulate these treatable risk factors. The incidence among hospitalized elderly is substantially higher and continues to be a risk factor for at least 1 mo after discharge [1].

APPROACH TO THE PATIENT

All patients >65 yrs, especially those with risk factors, should be screened frequently by being asked specifically about falls or near-falls. Patients may be reluctant to volunteer this information because of fear of institutionalization. Modifiable risk factors should be addressed before the first fall for at-risk patients. **Two falls in a 6-mo period or any fall resulting in serious injury should trigger a complete evaluation and multicomponent intervention.**

The evaluation should include key components of the history and physical exam, review of medications, identification of environmental and situational factors, cognitive assessment, performance assessment, and recognition of acute illnesses.

HISTORY

The history should first focus on the exact circumstances of the fall. Information from witnesses may be helpful. Symptoms of dysequilibrium should be sought and are discussed elsewhere in this text (see Chap. 8, Dizziness, Syncope, and Orthostatic Hypotension). The pneumonic **CATASTROPHE** can be used to identify other key components of the history (Table 7-2).

MEDICATION REVIEW

Evaluation of falls is always a good time to review medications and try to address issues of inappropriate drug prescribing or polypharmacy (see Chap. 6, Approach to Polypharmacy and Appropriate Medication Use). Medications that may **increase the risk of falling** include the following:

• Sedative-hypnotics, particularly benzodiazepines and zolpidem (Ambien)

TABLE 7-2. CATASTROPHE: A MNEMONIC FOR OBTAINING
A HISTORY AFTER A FALL

C—Caregiver and housing	T—Teetering (dizziness)
A—Alcohol (including withdrawal)	R—Recent illness (or hospitalization)
T—Treatment (medications, including compliance)	O—Ocular problems
	P—Pain with mobility
A—Affect (depression or lack of initiative)	H—Hearing
S—Syncope	E—Environmental hazards

From Sloan JP. Mobility failure. In: *Protocols in primary care geriatrics.* New York: Springer,
1997:33–38, with permission.

* Antidepressants
* Antiemetics
* Anticholinergic drugs, including antihistamines
* Antihypertensives and vasodilators
* NSAIDs
* Hypoglycemic agents
* Antipsychotics
* Calcium-channel blockers

PHYSICAL EXAM

The physical exam should focus on acute processes, orthostatic BP measurement, sensory function, motor exam, cognitive function, foot problems, and performance assessment. **The mnemonic I HATE FALLING can be a useful tool for remembering the key components of the exam** (Table 7-3).

If the patient is able to stand from a sitting position with his or her arms folded across the chest, then he or she is asked to repeat the task five times as fast as possible. Times >10 secs suggest the presence of lower extremity proximal muscle weakness [2]. **Gait is assessed by asking the patient to walk 12 ft at his or her normal pace, turn, and return without stopping.** The number of steps required to traverse 12 ft and the number of steps required to turn 180 degrees provides a quantitative measure of dynamic balance. This test is a useful tool for identification of ataxia, stride variability, gait instability, and lower extremity weakness. The task can be repeated with the distraction of counting backward from 20 while the patient walks. The disparity between the times of the two gait assess-

TABLE 7-3. I HATE FALLING: A MNEMONIC FOR PHYSICAL
EXAMINATION OF THE PATIENT WITH FALLS

I—Inflammation of joints (or deformity)	F—Foot problems
H—Hypotension (orthostatic measurements)	A—Arrhythmia or valvular disease
A—Auditory and visual abnormalities	L—Leg-length discrepancy
T—Tremor (or other signs of parkinsonism)	L—Lack of conditioning (generalized weakness)
E—Equilibrium or balance (Romberg or pull-test)	I—Illness
	N—Nutritional status
	G—Gait disturbance

From Sloan JP. Mobility failure. In: *Protocols in primary care geriatrics.* New York: Springer,
1997:33–38, with permission.

ments is a measure of the patient's risk of falls. **The Progressive Romberg is a quantita-tive measure of static balance** [3]. The patient is asked to stand for 10 secs with eyes open and then closed in three different positions: feet together (Romberg stance), one foot halfway in front of the other (semi-tandem stance), and then with the heel of one foot against the toe of the other (tandem stance). The score is the number of stances success-fully maintained for 10 secs (see Chap. 1, Approach to the Geriatric Patient: Comprehensive Geriatric Assessment, for scoring sheet). The time to say the months of the year in reverse order is a simple measure of the speed of processing sensory information, a major risk factor for falls.

DIAGNOSTIC WORKUP

Further workup should be individualized and may include measurement of 25-OH vitamin D, intact PTH, vitamin B_{12}, electrolytes, drug levels, and thyroid function tests. Findings may also warrant ECG, Holter monitor, bone density assessment, and brain imaging studies.

INTERVENTIONS

The goals of intervention should be to decrease the risk of falls, decrease the risk of injury from falls, reduce fear of falling, and prolong functional independence. Just as the cause of falls is frequently multifactorial, recent clinical trials prove that **multifacto-rial interventions** are the most effective means to decrease falls and fear of falls [4]. Once the interventions are initiated, they should be continued indefinitely to maintain benefit.

Exercise programs are encouraged for older people and should include strength, endurance, and balance training [5]. Recent research suggests that Tai Chi is a useful method of balance training [6]. Home therapy may be an option for homebound patients.

Environmental modifications include raised toilet seats, clearing the home of clutter and obstacles, handrails, improved lighting, appropriate footwear, and nonslip surfaces. Throw rugs should be removed. **A home safety evaluation, typically provided by occu-pational thereapy, provides information and patient education regarding correctable safety issues within the home.**

Medication reviews should be performed with emphasis on the goal of eliminating polypharmacy. Contributing drugs should be discontinued. (See Chap. 6, Approach to Polypharmacy and Appropriate Medication Use.)

Gait retraining is useful to instruct patients in correct gait and appropriate use of assistive devices such as canes and walkers.

Physical therapy is recommended for patients with generalized or focal weakness. The physical therapy consult should entail a gait assessment and lower extremity strength training exercises.

Treatment of comorbid conditions that predispose to greater risk of injurious falls is an integral component of a fall intervention program.

Osteoporosis should be identified and treated with calcium and vitamin D, hormone replacement therapy, and antiresorptive medications as appropriate (see Chap. 14, Osteoporosis). However, it is worth noting that a fall from standing height generates more than sufficient force to cause a fracture in elderly patients with average bone density.

Hip protectors have recently been shown to significantly reduce the risk of fracture due to falls [7]. Currently, none of the studied devices are available in the United States.

Nutritional status should be assessed and corrected as possible.

Provide **Lifeline** alert or related systems for patients at risk for falling who will spend any time alone.

FALLS IN THE HOSPITAL

Falls occur more often in the hospital than in the community, likely because of acute illnesses, dehydration, medications, and delirium. Management should consist of identifying patients at risk and preventing falls before they happen. **Restraints and bed rails do not prevent falls and may cause more serious injuries.** Bed alarms may help alert staff that a patient is trying to get out of bed without the use of restraints or bed rails. **Many patients fall trying to get out of bed for legitimate reasons, so timed toileting and adequate access to food and water should be provided.** Delirium should be assessed and managed appropriately (see Chap. 4, Delirium). Using single, quiet rooms is preferable. **Avoid inappropriate sedatives and sleepers.** Many of these interventions are incorporated into dedicated geriatric inpatient units, such as the acute care for the elderly unit (see Chap. 2, Settings for Geriatric Care).

KEY POINTS TO REMEMBER

- Falling is a serious and common condition in the elderly that results in functional decline, loss of independence, institutionalization, and serious injury.
- The etiology of most falls is multifactorial, but many of the factors can be modified.
- Patients >65 yrs, particularly those with risk factors for fall or a history of falling, should undergo appropriate evaluation to prevent falls.
- A fall workup should include a review of medications and elimination of polypharmacy and inappropriate medications when possible.
- Fall prevention is best achieved with a multicomponent intervention to address modifiable factors.

SUGGESTED READING

Birge SJ. Can falls and hip fractures be prevented in frail older adults? *J Am Geriatr Soc* 1999;47:1265–1266.

Cutson TM. Falls in the elderly. *Am Fam Phys* 1994;49:149–156.

Feder F, Cryer C, Donovan S, et al. Guidelines for the prevention of falls in people over 65. *BMJ* 2000;321:1007–1011.

Fuller GF. Falls in the elderly. *Am Fam Phys* 2000,01.2159–2160.

Hanger H, Ball MC, Wood LA. An analysis of falls in the hospital: can we do without bedrails? *J Am Geriatr Soc* 1999;47:529–531.

King MB, Tinetti ME. A multifactorial approach to reducing injurious falls. *Clin Geriatr Med* 1996;12:745–759.

Podsiadlo D, Richardson S. The timed "up and go": a test of basic functional mobility for frail elderly persons. *J Am Geriatr Soc* 1991;39:142–148.

Sloan JP. Mobility failure. In: *Protocols in primary care geriatrics*. New York: Springer, 1997:33–38.

REFERENCES

1. Mahoney JE, Palta M, Johnson J, et al. Temporal association between hospitalization and rate of falls after discharge. *Arch Intern Med* 2000;160:2788–2795.
2. Csuka M, McCarty DJ. Simple method for measurement of lower extremity muscle strength. *Am J Med* 1985;78:77–81.
3. Guralnik JM, Simonsick EM, Ferrucci L, et al. A short physical performance battery assess lower extremity function: association with self-reported disability and prediction of mortality and nursing home admission. *J Gerontol Med Sci* 1998;49:M85–M94.
4. Tinetti ME, et al. A multifactorial intervention to reduce the risk of falling among elderly people living in the community. *N Engl J Med* 1994;331:821–827.
5. Robertson MC, Devlin N, Gardner MM, et al. Effectiveness and economic evaluation of a nurse delivered home exercise programme to prevent falls. 1: Randomized controlled trial. *BMJ* 2001;322:697–701.
6. Wu G. Evaluation of the effectiveness of Tai Chi for improving balance and preventing falls in the older population—a review. *J Am Geriatr Soc* 2002;50:746–754.
7. Kannus P, Parkkari J, Niemi S, et al. Prevention of hip fracture in elderly people with use of a hip protector. *N Engl J Med* 2000;343:1506–1513.

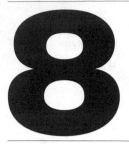

Dizziness, Syncope, and Orthostatic Hypotension

Roger Kerzner

INTRODUCTION

Dizziness, syncope, and orthostatic hypotension are presented together because there is substantial overlap in how patients present and in the etiologies and treatments for these conditions. **Distinguishing among these three syndromes is the first step in their management.** Questioning will usually distinguish dizziness (vertigo or sense of spinning or motion) from syncope, near-syncope (lightheadedness, complete or near loss of consciousness), and orthostasis (unsteadiness or lightheadedness after changes in position). It is particularly important to ask about these symptoms in patients who have fallen (see Chap. 7, Falls).

DIZZINESS

Sensations of motion while standing, lightheadedness, and imbalance are common problems in older persons that are often described as dizziness. Aging predisposes to this condition through diminished capacity in the vestibular system, vision, and proprioception [1]. Although the prevalence ranges between 13–38% of elderly individuals, it should not be attributed to normal aging, and an underlying diagnosis or multiple diagnoses should be sought [2].

Differential Diagnosis

Categorizing the symptom of dizziness is a useful way to uncover an underlying diagnosis (Table 8-1) [1,3]. Unfortunately, only one-half of elderly patients can be placed in one subtype. Some authors have suggested that dizziness should be considered a "geriatric syndrome" with multiple etiologies [2] that need to be discovered.

Vertigo
Vertigo, **a sensation of spinning or motion,** usually arises from the vestibular system in either the ear or brain. Common causes are benign positional vertigo, cerebrovascular disease, and acute labyrinthitis/vestibular neuronitis. Other possibilities include otitis media, some drug toxicities (i.e., aminoglycosides), and panic disorder.

Presyncopal Lightheadedness
Presyncopal lightheadedness, **or the sensation of almost fainting,** predominantly results from cerebral hypoperfusion. This includes orthostatic hypotension, cardiac arrhythmias, congestive heart failure, and vasovagal episodes.

Dysequilibrium
Dysequilibrium, **the feeling of imbalance or unsteadiness, is generally a nonspecific description of dizziness resulting from any disturbance of the motor control system.** Classically, neuromuscular diseases, cerebellar diseases, and stroke are considered. Uniquely common causes in older persons include physical deconditioning and multiple neurosensory deficits such as visual impairment, vestibular dysfunction, and mild peripheral neuropathy that combine to cause unsteadiness.

TABLE 8-1. DIFFERENTIAL DIAGNOSIS OF DIZZINESS IN THE ELDERLY

Vertigo	Congestive heart failure
Benign positional vertigo	Vasovagal episodes
Cerebrovascular disease	**Dysequilibrium**
Acute labyrinthitis/vestibular neuronitis	Neuromuscular diseases Stroke
Otitis media	Cerebellar diseases
Drug toxicities	Physical deconditioning
Ménière's disease	Multiple neurosensory deficits
Cervical dizziness	**Panic disorder and other psychological diseases**
Acoustic neuroma	
Presyncopal lightheadedness	
Orthostatic hypotension	
Cardiac arrhythmias	

Evaluation

A thorough history is important to determine the subtype of dizziness and subsequent diagnosis. The key is to identify critical diagnoses with serious morbidity and to be mindful of the variety of diagnostic possibilities. Some techniques for accomplishing this include the following:

* Evaluate for **life-threatening conditions** that are generally rare causes of dizziness, such as a stroke or ischemic heart disease.
* Concentrate on the **temporal pattern** of the dizziness. Continuous dizziness is associated with degenerative or psychological diseases or results from permanent damage like a stroke. In patients with episodic dizziness, the duration of the episodes is important. **Benign positional vertigo lasts <1 min, transient ischemic attacks between 20 mins and 2 hrs, and Ménière's disease episodes last 2 hrs to 2 days.**
* **Identify comorbid illnesses and obtain a detailed drug history.** Cervical osteoarthritis frequently causes dizziness through compression of the vestibular arteries or stimulation of proprioceptive centers with neck positioning. Medications to consider include those for cardiovascular diseases; drugs with anticholinergic properties, including meclizine; and psychotropics. One should also inquire about alcohol, caffeine, and over-the-counter drugs such as cold preparations and sleeping pills, which often cause dizziness.
* In the **physical exam,** emphasize the neurologic exam and perform provocative maneuvers to elicit vertigo (Dick-Hallpike maneuver). Eye movements should be closely evaluated for nystagmus.
* **Lab testing** and **imaging** should be used in a directed manner, as they often have low yield [1].

Treatment

Treatment should focus on the etiology of the dizziness, but for many patients a specific diagnosis cannot be identified. Alternatively, most cases are benign and self-limited, and dizziness is not associated with excess mortality in older persons [1]. It is associated with increased risk for falls and functional disability; thus, multidimensional interventions should be applied in most patients regardless of the diagnosis [2].

- **Exercise and activity programs** to provide strengthening and gait training should be prescribed. Involving a physical therapist with these goals can be very beneficial. For patients with chronic vestibular disease, therapists can teach specific vestibular desensitization exercises (Epley maneuver).
- Consider having the patient use a **cane or walker.**
- **Correct visual impairment.**
- **Eliminate contributing medications.**
- Aggressively **treat comorbid depression and anxiety,** which can magnify the impact of dizziness.
- Make the home hazard free by installing night-lights and arranging for a **home assessment** by an occupational therapist.
- **Meclizine (Antivert) is rarely helpful** for these syndromes and may contribute to cognitive dysfunction and fall risk in the elderly.

SYNCOPE

Syncope is a sudden loss of consciousness associated with a loss of postural tone, followed by spontaneous recovery. In older persons, age-related changes predispose to syncopal events. This includes changes in the heart that lead to hypotension if preload is decreased, decreased baroreflex sensitivity and cerebral blood flow, and impaired thirst mechanisms with a diminished renal capacity to conserve sodium, which contributes to dehydration. Syncope is thus extremely common in older persons, occurring in >10% of nursing home residents each year [4].

Differential Diagnosis

Cardiovascular
Elderly persons are particularly susceptible to arrhythmic syncope, especially sinus node disease and atrioventricular block from degeneration of the conduction system (Table 8-2). A serious but uncommon cardiac cause of syncope is a myocardial infarction (MI). In a study of nursing home patients, 10% of patients with MI presented with syncope [5]. Other cardiogenic causes include aortic stenosis, hypertrophic cardiomyopathy, aortic dissection, and, indirectly, pulmonary embolism. Carotid sinus syncope primarily occurs in older persons with coronary artery disease, HTN, and neck problems and should be considered in older persons with unexplained syncope.

Noncardiovascular
Orthostatic hypotension (see below) is a particularly common problem in older persons secondary to age-related changes, volume depletion, and comorbid medical conditions

TABLE 8-2. DIFFERENTIAL DIAGNOSIS OF SYNCOPE IN THE ELDERLY

Cardiovascular	Noncardiovascular
Tachy- and bradyarrhythmias	Neurocardiogenic/vasovagal (e.g., fecal impaction, bowel obstruction, urinary retention)
Myocardial infarction	
Aortic stenosis	Orthostatic hypotension, including postprandial hypotension
Hypertrophic cardiomyopathy	
Carotid sinus syncope; in older persons with coronary artery disease, HTN, and neck problems	Medications (antihypertensives, antiarrhythmics, digoxin, psychoactive medications, alcohol)
Pulmonary embolism, indirectly	Coexistent medical illness (e.g., UTI, pneumonia, and medications)
Aortic dissection	Cerebrovascular disease
	Psychiatric; less common in the elderly

such as diabetes, infection, and medications. **Common medications that can contribute to orthostasis include almost all antihypertensive agents, antiarrhythmics, digoxin, some psychoactive drugs, and alcohol.** A variant of orthostatic hypotension is postprandial hypotension, which may be present in up to a quarter of nursing home residents [5]. Other noncardiovascular causes include neurocardiogenic or vasovagal syncope and cerebrovascular disease. The interaction of a coexistent medical illness such as a UTI, pneumonia, and medications can also lead to syncope. Psychiatric causes of syncope are more common in younger patients [6].

Evaluation

Older patients should be admitted to the hospital for evaluation of their syncope because of the high frequency of serious underlying diagnoses. Whereas a single predominating cause usually leads to the clinical event, it is important to recognize that in older patients, multiple factors and comorbidities usually contribute and should be identified.

History

A careful clinical history has the highest diagnostic yield for identifying the cause of syncope [7]. The first step is to clarify the scenario of the syncopal event by interviewing the patient, his or her family, and any other witnesses. This is done to determine whether an actual episode of syncope occurred as opposed to dizziness, vertigo, or a seizure. Dizziness and vertigo are not associated with a loss of consciousness. A sensation of aura before the event or slowness in recovering consciousness (>5 mins) is associated with seizures. Rhythmic movements or jerks can be seen with either syncope or a seizure [6]. Alternatively, a significant number of elderly patients evaluated for unexplained dizziness or falls will have diagnoses more often associated with syncope, such as carotid-sinus hypersensitivity [8].

Once the syncopal event has been defined, identifying symptoms and behavior from the preceding minutes to days is useful. Symptoms that occur after standing or eating a meal indicate orthostatic or postprandial hypotension. Chest pain, palpitations, or dyspnea might suggest ischemia, arrhythmias, or a pulmonary embolus. **A prodrome of nausea, diaphoresis, or flushing or an identified emotional or situational trigger is associated with neurocardiogenic syncope. On the other hand, the lack of prodromal symptoms in a patient with heart disease suggests an arrhythmia.** Inquiring about oral intake, last bowel movement, and signs of an infection such as fever, cough, or dysuria in the preceding days is important to uncover the multiple factors that led to the event. Finally, **a thorough review of the patient's medications is necessary.**

Physical Exam

The three key features of a full exam are an assessment of orthostatic vital signs and careful cardiovascular and neurologic exams. The cardiovascular exam should be directed to uncover structural heart disease, because this is a predictor of mortality in patients with syncope [6]. Carotid-sinus massage can be performed but is contraindicated in patients with a carotid bruit.

Diagnostic Testing

As the etiology of a syncopal event is often multifactorial, a thorough evaluation is indicated in all patients. Diagnostic testing should not be stopped simply because a single contributing diagnosis, such as a UTI, is identified in the early parts of the evaluation. It may be appropriate, however, to treat some of the initial contributing causes of a syncopal event before pursuing invasive testing.

Baseline Lab Testing

Baseline lab testing of **electrolytes, renal function, and a UA** are indicated in all older patients to discover contributing illnesses, although they rarely reveal the only cause of a syncopal event.

ECG
ECGs often have abnormalities that provide clues to a diagnosis but are rarely diagnostic by themselves.

24-Hour Ambulatory ECG Monitoring
As older patients should be admitted to a hospital to evaluate any episode of syncope, monitoring for 24 hrs can be easily performed in all patients to correlate symptoms with an arrhythmia or lack of one. Extending the monitoring >24 hrs does not substantially increase the yield of the monitoring [5].

Echocardiogram
When the presence of structural heart disease is difficult to determine clinically, an echocardiogram can be useful. This is particularly true for valvular lesions that cannot be confidently characterized with auscultation alone. Structural abnormalities that are discovered may not necessarily explain the syncopal event [9].

Chemistry Testing for Myocardial Infarction
Chemistry testing for an MI is indicated in all older patients. Testing for a MI in the setting of syncope should not automatically trigger empiric treatment for an acute coronary syndrome. For instance, beta blockers might precipitate bradycardia that could have contributed to the original syncopal episode.

Invasive Electrophysiologic Studies
Invasive electrophysiologic studies should be considered in elderly patients with structural heart disease, ECG abnormalities, and unexplained syncope. Consultation with a specialist is recommended because of the difficulty in diagnosing unexplained syncope in elderly patients.

Tilt-Table Testing
Tilt-table testing should be considered for patients with a normal ECG and no heart disease. Consultation with a specialist is recommended because of the difficulty in diagnosing unexplained syncope in elderly patients.

Carotid Sinus Massage
Performing carotid sinus massage in a monitored setting is useful for patients with symptoms associated with turning of the head or shaving or recurrent syncope with an otherwise negative evaluation.

Neurologic Testing
EEGs and cranial imaging have a low diagnostic yield unless a patient has a history consistent with a seizure.

Treatment
Treatment is directed at the underlying diagnosis. As mentioned earlier (p. 45), it may be appropriate to treat some of the initial contributing causes of a syncopal event before pursuing invasive testing. Regardless of the medical management, instructions on measures to prevent repercussions of syncopal events are important. This includes avoidance of driving, arranging a home safety evaluation to avoid an injury from a fall, other fall precautions (treatment of osteoporosis and use of hip pads), and avoidance of Foley catheters that could contribute to UTIs.

Orthostatic and Postprandial Hypotension
See Orthostatic Hypotension.

Neurocardiogenic Syncope
There is limited evidence supporting a particular strategy for treating neurocardiogenic syncope, especially in older persons. Atenolol and paroxetine may be beneficial [6].

TABLE 8-3. DIFFERENTIAL DIAGNOSIS OF ORTHOSTATIC HYPOTENSION

Hypovolemia	Alcohol
Poor food and fluid intake	Antiparkinsonian agents
Overdiuresis	**Primary autonomic neuropathies**
GI losses (vomiting, diarrhea)	Parkinson's disease
Adrenal insufficiency	Multiple system atrophy
Medications	**Secondary autonomic neuropathies**
Diuretics	Uremia
Antihypertensives	Diabetes mellitus
Antiarrhythmics	Alcoholism
Digoxin	Vitamin B_{12} deficiency
Psychotropic medications	**Postprandial hypotension**

ORTHOSTATIC HYPOTENSION

Orthostatic hypotension, a fall in SBP of at least 20 mm Hg or to <90 mm Hg with standing, is a particularly common problem in older persons. The prevalence ranges from 8–24% in the general elderly population and up to 50% in nursing home residents [5,10]. The etiology is often multifactorial. This includes age-related changes like decreased baroreceptor reflex sensitivity and loss of arterial compliance and comorbid medical conditions and the medications used to treat them. **If orthostasis is suspected, BP should be measured in the supine, sitting, and standing positions on repeated occasions (after medications, after meals, etc.).** Document the pulse, BP, circumstances, and presence of symptoms.

Differential Diagnosis

Table 8-3 lists the differential diagnosis of orthostatic hypotension.

Treatment

As with syncope and dizziness, treatment should be directed at the underlying etiology. Other strategies to consider include the following [5]:

- **Discontinue contributing medications if possible.**
- **Avoid situations that may exacerbate orthostasis** such as standing motionless or prolonged recumbency, large meals, hot weather, and hot showers.
- **Elevate the head of the bed** to stimulate the renin-angiotensin-aldosterone system.
- **Wear waist-high support stockings.**
- **For exercise, consider swimming because hydrostatic pressure opposes the gravitational effect on blood pooling.**
- **Increase salt and fluid intake of patients without congestive heart failure.**
- **Drug therapy:** If nonpharmacologic methods are unsuccessful, medications may need to be instituted to prevent injuries. Risk of treatment-related supine HTN must be balanced against the benefit obtained in reducing symptomatic orthostatic hypotension.
    - Caffeine, 100 mg with meals or 1 cup of coffee.
    - Fludrocortisone (Florinef), 0.1 mg PO qd–tid.
    - Midodrine (ProAmatine), 2.5–5 mg PO tid.

POSTPRANDIAL HYPOTENSION

A common variant of orthostatic hypotension is postprandial hypotension. It may be present in up to one-fourth of nursing home residents and has been correlated with syncope, falls, new coronary events, stroke, and total mortality [4]. **It can be managed by eating many small meals rather than large ones, decreasing the sugar content of the meal, avoiding alcohol, minimizing exercise after meals, and avoiding medications that predispose to orthostatic hypotension.** Caffeine given with meals may be beneficial.

KEY POINTS TO REMEMBER

- Sensations of motion, lightheadedness, imbalance, and syncope are common problems in older adults that are commonly described as dizziness.
- A thorough history is important to determine which syndrome the patient is describing (vertigo, syncope, near-syncope, dysequilibrium, orthostasis). It is also the best way to diagnose the underlying etiology (vasodepressor, cardiogenic, seizure).
- Adjunctive history from witnesses of events can be invaluable.
- The elderly should be admitted to the hospital for evaluation of syncope because of the higher incidence of serious underlying diagnoses.
- Orthostatic hypotension is a common problem that may be related to medications, volume depletion, autonomic dysfunction, alcohol, and postprandial hypotension.
- Treatment is individualized based on the underlying causes, which may be multiple.

SUGGESTED READING

Furman JM, Cass SP. Benign paroxysmal positional vertigo. *N Engl J Med* 1999;341: 1590–1596.

Schaal SF. Syncope in the elderly. In: Wenger NK, ed. *Cardiovascular disease in the octogenarian and beyond*. London: Martin Dunitz, 1999:93–110.

REFERENCES

1. Sloan PD. Evaluation and management of dizziness in the older patient. *Clin Geriatr Med* 1996;12:785–801.
2. Tinetti ME, Williams CS, Gill TM. Dizziness among older adults: a possible geriatric syndrome. *Ann Intern Med* 2000;132:337–344.
3. Drachman D, Hart C. An approach to the dizzy patient. *Neurology* 1972;22:323–334.
4. Aronow WS, Ahn C. Association of postprandial hypotension with incidence of falls, syncope, coronary events, stroke, and total mortality at 29-month follow-up of 499 older nursing home residents. *J Am Geriatr Soc* 1995;45:1015.
5. Aronow WS. Dizziness and syncope. In: Hazzard WR, ed. *Principles of geriatric medicine and gerontology*, 4th ed. New York: McGraw-Hill, 1999:1519–1534.
6. Kapoor WN. Syncope. *N Engl J Med* 2000;343:1856–1862.
7. Linzer M, Yang EH, Estes NA III, et al. Diagnosing syncope. 1. Value of history, physical examination, and electrocardiography: Clinical Efficacy Assessment Project of the American College of Physicians. *Ann Intern Med* 1997;126:989–996.
8. McIntosh SJ, Lawson J, Kenny RA. Clinical characteristics of vasopressor, cardioinhibitory, and mixed carotid sinus syndrome in the elderly. *Am J Med* 1993; 95:203–208.
9. Recchia D, Barzilai B. Echocardiography in the evaluation of patients with syncope. *J Gen Intern Med* 1995;10:649–655.
10. Ooi WL, Hossain M, Lipsitz LA. The association between orthostatic hypotension and recurrent falls in nursing home residents. *Am J Med* 2000;108:106–111.

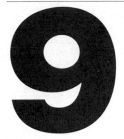

Unintentional Weight Loss in the Elderly

Randall Wooley

INTRODUCTION

Part of any geriatric assessment and longitudinal care should be attentive to the patient's weight and any change in weight over time. There are several reasons for weight loss in elderly patients, and there may be multiple causes in any given patient. The definition of involuntary weight loss is a loss of 1–2%/wk, 5%/mo, or 10% in a 6-mo period. **An unintentional weight loss is associated with increased mortality in elderly patients.**

POTENTIAL CAUSES

The multiple causes of weight loss include physical, emotional, and social factors. The "MEALS ON WHEELS" mnemonic serves as a guide to evaluating weight loss (Table 9-1). **Some of the most common diagnoses include depression, malignancy, GI disorders, thyroid dysfunction, and side effects from medications.**

PRESENTATION

History

Questioning should be broad to encompass the numerous potential etiologies:

- Obtain **collateral information** from a caregiver or relative.
- Ask how the patient obtains and prepares food, including financial difficulties in obtaining food.
- Inquire about any difficulties in using utensils, chewing, or swallowing.
- Assess for any changes in appetite (see Appendix F for an appetite questionnaire and nutrition screen).
- Ask about **specific types and amounts of food consumed,** and estimate daily caloric intake. Is there a schedule for eating or regular snacks?
- A **medication history** is vital, as certain medications can affect taste and appetite.
  - ACE inhibitors can cause dysgeusia.
  - Digoxin and SSRIs can suppress appetite.
  - Anticholinergic and antihistaminic drugs can cause dry mouth and difficulty swallowing.
- Determine whether there is any **abdominal pain or postprandial nausea,** which may represent mesenteric ischemia or biliary, pancreatic, or gastric disease.
- The patient should be **screened for depression** (see Chap. 5, Depression in the Older Adult, and Appendix C). A positive screening test should be followed up with a complete evaluation for depression.
- Assess contribution of **comorbidities** such as severe heart failure (cardiac cachexia), malignancy, or COPD.

Physical Exam

For every elderly patient, **weight should be checked at every visit and compared with previous weights.** If weights are unavailable, determine whether the patient's

TABLE 9-1. MEALS ON WHEELS MNEMONIC FOR ETIOLOGIES OF UNINTENTIONAL WEIGHT LOSS IN THE ELDERLY

M — Medication effects, malignancy

E — Emotional problems, depression

A — Anorexia, alcoholism

L — Late-life paranoia

S — Swallowing and esophageal disorders

O — Oral factors (caries, ill-fitted dentures, dry mouth)

N — No money

W — Wandering (dementia-related behavior)

H — Hyper-/hypothyroidism, hyperparathyroidism, hypoadrenalism, hypogonadism, hyperglycemia

E — Enteric problems, including gastritis, ulcers, and malabsorption

E — Eating problems (unable to feed self)

L — Low-salt, low-cholesterol diets

S — Social problems, shopping (isolation, inability to obtain or prepare food)

---

clothes are fitting more loosely or clothing size has changed. Document the patient's weight and BMI. Observe for depressed mood and affect. Examine the oral cavity for oral ulcers, dentition, stomatitis, thrush, and poorly fitting dentures. Perform an abdominal exam to assess for tenderness, and perform a rectal exam to assess for occult blood loss, impaction, or mass.

Lab Studies

Basic lab studies should include a **CBC, measurement of electrolytes and renal function, liver enzymes, albumin, cholesterol, TSH, and UA.** Use of a dietary log and calorie counts may be useful. Additional studies can be ordered based on any observed abnormalities. Circumstances may require further diagnostic studies such as CT scans, endoscopy, swallowing evaluation, or evaluation for micronutrient deficiencies.

MANAGEMENT

The treatment of unintentional weight loss should be directed at the underlying disorder.

Counsel the patient and meal providers/caregivers regarding nutritional needs.

For community-dwelling patients, **meals-on-wheels programs** can help provide a daytime meal when caregivers are at work or need help. Most **geriatric day programs** also provide meals.

Nutritional support should be provided with supplements (if the patient is able to swallow). Carnation Instant Breakfast is a relatively cheap dietary supplement available in many flavors. It is added to milk and provides 1–1.5 calories/mL. Consider adding a daily multivitamin. Enteral or parenteral nutrition may need to be considered.

Remove excessive dietary restrictions (renal, diabetic, or low-sodium diets) to make meals more palatable.

Provide foods of the needed consistency and ensure proper-fitting dentalwear.

Treat underlying disorders, including depression, constipation and other GI disorders, heart failure, and lung disease.

Remove offending medications.

After trying nonpharmacologic interventions, medications may also be used. No drugs are currently FDA approved for the treatment of geriatric anorexia:

- **Megestrol** (Megace) may stimulate appetite and produces weight gain in some patients. Beneficial effects on weight and appetite have been observed in cancer, AIDS, and long-term care patients [1,2].
  - Dosing: start at 200 mg PO qd. The dose can be increased to 800 mg PO qd.
  - Adverse reactions: edema, vaginal bleeding, nausea, adrenal suppression, dyspnea (respiratory alkalosis), somnolence, cognitive impairment, and psychosis.
- **Dronabinol** (Marinol) is a synthetic cannabinoid that has been shown to improve appetite in cancer and AIDS patients [3]. It is effective for chemotherapy-induced nausea and vomiting [4].
  - Dosing: start 2.5 mg qd. Dose can be titrated up by 2.5-mg increments to 10 mg PO tid.
  - Adverse reactions: delirium, cognitive impairment, euphoria.
- **Mirtazapine** (Remeron) is an antidepressant that has been shown to increase appetite and weight when used in the treatment of depression [5]. Because SSRIs can be associated with anorexia and weight loss, some authorities consider it to be first-line treatment for depressed patients with significant weight loss.
  - Dosing: start 7.5–15 mg PO nightly. The dose can be increased q1–2wks up to 45 mg PO nightly.
  - Adverse reactions: most common are somnolence, constipation, and xerostomia.
- **Testosterone replacement therapy** should be considered for hypogonadal men (see Chap. 12, Androgen Deficiency in Older Men).
- **Oxymetholone** (Oxandrolone) is an anabolic-androgenic steroid that may stimulate weight gain and could be considered for selected men or women.

Follow-Up

The patient's dietary intake, appetite, and weight should be checked at every visit. Follow-up assessments should focus on continued investigation for underlying causes and monitoring the response to interventions.

KEY POINTS TO REMEMBER

- Unintentional weight loss in the elderly is associated with an increased mortality.
- Weight loss in the elderly is frequently multifactorial.
- The mnemonic MEALS ON WHEELS can help to recall the common causes of unintentional weight loss.
- A focused history can identify potential contributing factors, illnesses, and medications.
- The workup should include evaluation and treatment of depression.
- Management is directed at the underlying disorder. Removing medical and social barriers to adequate nutrition is essential.
- Pharmacologic therapy is an option, but long-term data are lacking.
- Unintentional weight loss in the elderly should always raise the possibility of malignancy.

SUGGESTED READING

Adelman AM, Daly MP. *20 Common problems in geriatrics*. New York: McGraw-Hill, 2001:338–348.

Gazewood JD, Mehr DR. Diagnosis and management of weight loss in the elderly. *J Fam Pract* 1998;47:19–25.

Ham RJ, Sloane PD, Warshaw GA. *Primary care geriatrics*. St. Louis: Mosby, 2002:122–127.

Huffman GB. Evaluating and treating unintentional weight loss in the elderly. *Am Fam Phys* 2002;65:640–650.

REFERENCES

1. Yeh SS, Wu SY, Lee TP, et al. Improvement in quality-of-life measures and stimulation of weight gain after treatment with megestrol acetate oral suspension in geriatric cachexia: results of a double-blind, placebo-controlled study. *J Am Geriatr Soc* 2000;48:485–492.

2. Von Roenn JH, Murphy RL, Wegener N. Megestrol acetate for treatment of anorexia and cachexia associated with human immunodeficiency virus infection. *Semin Oncol* 1990;17:13–16.
3. Beal JE, Olson R, Laubenstein L, et al. Dronabinol as a treatment for anorexia associated with weight loss in patients with AIDS. *J Pain Symptom Manage* 1995; 10:89–97.
4. Tramer MR, Carroll D, Campbell FA, et al. Cannabinoids for control of chemotherapy induced nausea and vomiting: quantitative systematic review. *BMJ* 2001;323: 16–21.
5. Benkert O, Szegedi A, Kohnen R. Mirtazapine compared with paroxetine in major depression. *J Clin Psychiatr* 2000;61:656–663.

10

Pressure Sores

Steve R. Lai

INTRODUCTION

Pressure ulcers are a serious and frequent occurrence among the elderly, especially those who are immobile and debilitated. There are an estimated 1.5–3 million Americans affected. **A pressure ulcer will develop in approximately 5% of patients admitted to acute care hospitals** [1]. Studies have shown that 60% of pressure ulcers develop in the hospital, 18% in the nursing home, and 18% at home [2]. In patients who undergo a hip fracture operation, one-third develop pressure ulcers. Pressure ulcers prolong the hospital stay, and the periop mortality rate is increased to 27% [3]. The prevalence of pressure ulcers in the long-term care setting is reported to be 15–25% at the time of admission [4]. Studies have shown that the longer the patient stays in a nursing home, the greater the likelihood that an ulcer will develop [5].

CAUSES

Pathophysiology

Pressure ulcers are localized areas of tissue necrosis that tend to occur when soft tissue is compressed between a bony prominence and external surface for a prolonged period [4]. The most common causes of wounds in older adults are pressure and friction. Other contributing factors include malnutrition, immobility, vascular insufficiency, and other systemic illnesses. Moisture from urinary or fecal incontinence, friction (pulling the patient across bed sheets), and shearing forces (patients sliding down a bed with the head elevated) can combine to further damage tissue.

PRESENTATION

Risk Factors

Extrinsic risk factors include pressure, shear (traction), and friction. **Intrinsic** risk factors include immobility, malnutrition, sensory loss, and moisture.

One of the most widely used scale to assess likelihood for development of pressure ulcers in individual patients is the **Norton scale** (Table 10-1; the Braden scale is also included in Appendix L). This scale assesses five factors: physical condition, mental condition, activity, mobility, and continence. Each of these factors is scored on a scale of 1–4. A total score of ≤ 16 is considered high risk and indicative of a need for preventive strategies [6].

Prevention

Prevention is the best treatment of pressure ulcers and is **essential for high-risk patients.** Table 10-2 gives guidelines for prevention of pressure ulcers.

Clinical Features

The development of pressure ulcers may lead to further problems, including osteomyelitis, cellulitis, infections of adjacent structures (e.g., joint spaces), bacteremia, and sepsis.

TABLE 10-1. NORTON SCALE USED TO ASSESS THE RISK OF DEVELOPING A PRESSURE ULCER [6]

Physical condition	Mental condition	Activity	Mobility	Incontinent
Good: 4	Alert: 4	Ambulant: 4	Full: 4	Not: 4
Fair: 3	Apathetic: 3	Walk/help: 3	Mildly limited: 3	Occasionally: 3
Poor: 2	Confused: 2	Confused: 2	Very limited: 2	Usually/urine: 2
Very bad: 1	Stupor: 1	Stupor: 1	Immobile: 1	Doubly: 1

Note: A total score of ≤ 16 indicated the patient is at high risk.
From Norton D, McLaren R, Exton-Smith AN. An investigation of geriatric nursing problems in hospitals. London: Churchill Livingstone, 1962, with permission.

Cellulitis may be difficult to diagnose in this setting because the ulcers will often have reactive hyperemia and erythema associated with normal healing. Findings that may suggest cellulitis include fever, enlarging ulcer, foul odor, and purulent drainage.

The evaluation for **osteomyelitis** is required when ulcers are clinically infected or nonhealing [4]. **Osteomyelitis has been detected in the bone underlying 26% of non-healing ulcers** [7]. Furthermore, osteomyelitis is difficult to diagnose because findings on soft tissue cultures, radiographic studies, and nuclear imaging studies are often abnormal in areas surrounding a pressure ulcer. MRI may be helpful in the diagnosis. An elevated ESR can suggest osteomyelitis but is a nonspecific test. The gold standard for diagnosis remains a bone biopsy [7].

Assessment

Once a pressure ulcer has been identified, the characteristics and stage should be noted (Table 10-3). Assessment may be difficult in patients with pigmented skin.

If an eschar is present, it should be removed by sharp débridement or with topical enzymatic agents (collagenase) to make an accurate assessment. Exposure of granulation tissue also facilitates healing.

The margins and depth of the wound should be explored with a sterile swab. If the wound tracks down to bone on exam, osteomyelitis is likely.

TABLE 10-2. GUIDELINES FOR PREVENTION OF PRESSURE ULCERS [8]

Mechanical loading and support surface guidelines
  For bed-bound persons
    Reposition at least q2h
    Use pillows or foam wedges to keep bony prominences from direct contact
    Use devices that relieve pressure on heels
    Avoid positioning directly on the trochanter
    Elevate the head of the bed as little as possible
    Use lifting devices to move rather than drag patients during transfers
    Use pressure-reducing mattress
Skin care and early treatment guidelines
  Inspect skin at least once a day
  Individualize bathing schedule, use moisturizers for dry skin
  Minimize environmental factors—low humidity and cold air
  Involve a multidisciplinary team when available

TABLE 10-3. STAGING OF PRESSURE ULCERS [9]

Stage I	Nonblanchable erythema of intact skin. Warmth, edema, induration, or hardness.
Stage II	Partial thickness skin loss involving the epidermis and/or dermis. Superficial ulcer, abrasion, blister, or shallow crater.
Stage III	Full-thickness skin loss involving damage to or necrosis of subcutaneous tissue that may extend down to, but not through, underlying fascia.
Stage IV	Full-thickness skin loss with extensive destruction, tissue necrosis, or damage to muscle, bone, or supporting structures (tendons, joint capsule).

For wounds on extremities, assess the vascular supply. Examine the peripheral pulses, capillary refill, coloration, and temperature. Arterial Doppler studies may help noninvasively assess for peripheral vascular disease.

Swab cultures of the wound surface often do not accurately identify causative organisms because the wound is often colonized with numerous organisms. For infected wounds, cultures can be useful for obtaining sensitivity data (infected wounds colonized with oxacillin-resistant *Staphylococcus aureus* may require vancomycin).

Assess nutritional status, including serum albumin. (See Chap. 9, Unintentional Weight Loss in the Elderly, and Appendix F.)

MANAGEMENT

Treatment

The treatment of pressure ulcers requires a comprehensive approach individualized for each patient. **The general principles are pressure reduction, control of infection, débridement, dressings, and nutritional support.**

Use a multidisciplinary skin care team when available. Wound care nurses, plastic surgeons, and other specialists can be an invaluable part of a team approach to wound care.

Pressure reduction is the top priority in treatment. Patients who are confined to bed should be turned every 2 hrs. In addition, a soft foam or air-waffle mattress should be used. For immobile patients or those with very large or multiple ulcers, an air-fluidized and low air-loss bed is the best option [10]. Other simple measures include pillows placed beneath calves and foam foot protection. Cushioning should be provided at bony prominences (between heels and knees or under trochanters). Patients should be scheduled to be out of bed as much as possible.

Stage II ulcers with a small amount of superficial necrotic tissue can be gently **débrided** mechanically with coarse mesh gauze moistened with saline, hydrocolloid dressings, or enzymatic débriding agents [4]. Stage III or IV ulcers are usually débrided surgically.

It is important to maintain a clean, moist **wound environment** to allow for optimal granulation and reepithelialization. A routinely changed wet-to-dry dressing can be used for dry, noninfected wounds. Excessive moisture can be managed with absorbent dressings (alginates) and reducing urinary and fecal incontinence (see Chap. 24, Urinary Incontinence). Scheduled toileting may help reduce soiling of involved areas. Foley catheters should be the last resort to keeping the environment clean.

There are six categories of **dressings**—gauze, films, foams, hydrocolloids, hydrogels, and alginate:

- Dressings and gels such as **hydrocolloids (DuoDERM, Tegasorb) and hydrogels (IntraSite, SoloSite) that cover the wound bed and provide a surface on which epithelial cells can migrate are often helpful for stage II or III wounds.**
- **Alginates are material derived from seaweed and are helpful in exudative wounds because they are very absorbent.**
- **Topical antibiotic creams are generally not used for routine wound care,** unless the area is infected or nonhealing.

Adequate **nutrition** is needed for normal wound healing. Protein or caloric supplementation may be indicated. There are some data to suggest **vitamin C and zinc sup-**

plementation may benefit refractory wound healing. Recommended doseages are vitamin C, 500 mg PO qd, and zinc sulfate, 220 mg PO qd.

IV antibiotics are used for pressure sores with associated cellulitis, deep tissue infection, or osteomyelitis. Topical antibiotics may help reduce bacterial counts.

Follow-Up

Wound care should not end at the time of discharge. Many patients will require continued aggressive care for months longer, either at home or in a long-term care facility. Home health can be arranged to provide skilled wound care, including dressing changes and serial assessments. Many centers have outpatient interdisciplinary wound clinics.

KEY POINTS TO REMEMBER

- Pressure and friction most commonly cause pressure sores.
- Most pressure sores occur in acute care settings, but many also develop at home or in long-term care facilities.
- The best treatment for pressure sores is prevention in high-risk patients. Risk can be assessed using the Norton scale.
- Multidisciplinary wound management teams should be involved when possible.
- Wound healing requires comprehensive management, including pressure unloading, shear reduction, mobilization, débridement, nutrition, dressings, and maintaining a clean, moist wound environment.

SUGGESTED READING

Allman RM, Laprade CA, Noel LB, et al. Pressure sores among hospitalized patients. *Ann Intern Med* 1986;105:337–342.

Carr DB. Geriatrics. In: Lin T, Rypkema S, eds. *The Washington manual of ambulatory therapeutics*. Philadelphia: Lippincott Williams & Wilkins, 2002:654–655.

Evans J, Andrews KL, Chutka DS, et al. Pressure ulcers: prevention and management. *Mayo Clinic Proc* 1995;70:789–799.

Sih R. Pressure ulcers in the nursing home. *Nursing Home Medicine* 1996;4:193–198.

REFERENCES

1. Allman RM. Epidemiology of pressure sores in different populations. *Decubitus* 1989;2:40–43.
2. Guralnik JM, Harris TB, White LR, et al. Occurrence and predictors of pressure sores in the National Health and Nutrition Examination survey follow-up. *J Am Geritr Soc* 1988;105:337–342.
3. Versluysen M. Pressure sores in elderly patients: the epidemiology related to hip operations. *J Bone Joint Surg Br* 1985;67:10–13.
4. Evans J, Andrews KL, Chutka DS, et al. Pressure ulcers: prevention and management. *Mayo Clinic Proc* 1995;70:789–799.
5. Brandeis GH, Morris JN, Nash DJ, et al. Incidence and healing rates of pressure ulcers in the nursing home. *Decubitus* 1989;2:60–62.
6. Norton D, McLaren RS, Exton-Smith AN. *Investigation of geriatric nursing problems in the hospital*. London: National Corporation for the Care of Old People, 1962.
7. Sugarman B. Pressure sores and underlying bone infection. *Arch Intern Med* 1987;147:553–555.
8. Panel for the Prediction of Pressure Ulcers in Adults. *Pressure ulcers in adults: prediction and prevention*. Clinical practice guideline, No. 3. Rockville, MD: Agency for Health Care Policy Research, 1992 (Publication No. AHCPR 92-1147).
9. National Pressure Ulcer Advisory Panel. Pressure ulcers prevalence, cost and risk assessment: consensus development conference statement. *Decubitus* 1989;2:24–28.
10. Ferrell BA, Osterweil D, Christenson P. A randomized trial of low-air-loss beds for treatment of pressure ulcers. *JAMA* 1993;269:494–497.

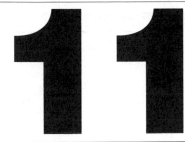

The Older Adult Driver

David B. Carr

INTRODUCTION

The automobile is the most important source of transportation for older adults. **The ability to drive or be driven is crucial for the elderly to maintain an important link with society.** Functional assessment, which can include driving ability, is a key component for clinicians involved in providing geriatric care. Clinicians should determine whether their patients are currently driving, provide information on healthy driving behaviors, assess medical conditions or physiologic variables that place their patient at risk for a motor vehicle injury or driving cessation, and treat medical illnesses that can impair driving skills.

The prevention of a motor vehicle crash is an appropriate goal for the primary care clinician. One could argue that impaired driving skill should not be viewed any different from the prevention, detection, and/or improvement of gait and balance disorders that can result in a fall or an unintentional injury.

CAUSES

Pathophysiology

Unintentional injury is now a leading cause of death in the United States [1]. Each year, motor vehicle crashes are associated with more than 40,000 deaths, 500,000 hospital admissions, 5,000,000 injuries, and a cost estimated to be $48.7 billion in lost productivity [2]. Older adults represent an increasing proportion of the motor vehicle injury problem each year. **Older adults are also more susceptible to injury in motor vehicle crashes than their younger counterparts** [3]. Epidemiologic studies have just begun to identify risk factors for driving cessation and motor vehicle crash and/or injury in older adults [4].

Human error is the most common cause for a motor vehicle crash. However, causes of motor vehicle crashes are not always obvious and may be complex. One study revealed that road user errors were present in 95% of accidents, and 44% of drivers were found to have made perceptual errors [5]. Perceptual errors included distraction, lack of attention, incorrect interpretation, misjudged speed and distance, and "looked, but failed to see." Crashes often result from human errors that may or may not be attributable to medical illness (i.e., visual impairment or alcohol use). There may be environmental and/or vehicular causes for any given crash that outweigh the contribution of impairment in driving skill.

PRESENTATION

Evaluation Process

Driving History

The assessment process should begin with the driving history. A checklist of important human, environmental, and vehicular factors to discuss with the patient and/or family can be found in Table 11-1. **It should be emphasized that obtaining history from a collateral source who has driven with the patient or observed his or her**

TABLE 11-1. IMPORTANT ASPECTS OF THE DRIVING HISTORY

Frequency, length, and reason for trips

Location (city vs. rural) of trips

Type of roadways used

Driving at night, rush hour, or adverse conditions

Use of a navigator

Presence of other caregivers that can drive

Familiarity with roadways

Caregivers' perception of driving skill

Transporting passengers

Crashes, tickets, near misses, lost while driving

From Carr DB. The older adult driver. *Am Fam Physician* 2000;61:141–146, with permission.

driving behavior is useful. Inquiries as to any close calls, mishaps, disorientation, or becoming lost in familiar areas should raise a red flag. **"Do you feel safe riding with the patient?"** can also be a useful question. If the answer is no, the interviewer should probe further to ask whether this is a "change." If the risky behavior has been noted for years, one should be reticent to attribute this change to a new medical illness.

Medical Conditions
There are relatively few studies that have focused on elderly drivers and medical conditions as risk factors for motor vehicle crashes. One study using a case control approach from a health maintenance organization found an increase in the crash and injury rate for **older diabetic patients taking insulin or hypoglycemic agents** [6]. A recent population-based study reported an increase in crashes and ticketed violations among older adults with **heart disease** [7]. Common diseases in older adult drivers that have been noted to affect driving ability include but are not limited to visual impairment [8], diabetes mellitus [9], seizure disorders [10], Alzheimer's disease [11], cerebrovascular accidents [12], depression [13], cardiovascular disease [14], sleep disorders [15], arthritis and related musculoskeletal disorders [16], and alcohol and drug use [17]. These are summarized in Table 11-2.

   Diseases should be graded as to their severity and ability to impact on driving errors or the "human factors." For instance, diabetes has a potential to affect the three important domains of driving: perception (retinopathy, cataract), cognition (hypoglycemia), and motor response (neuropathy). Thus, a clinician may have to make a determination as to the severity of the disease and weigh this finding with the set of patient characteristics (noncompliance). This becomes more difficult in older

TABLE 11-2. MEDICAL CONDITIONS ASSESSED BY PRIMARY CARE PHYSICIANS THAT MAY AFFECT DRIVING ABILITY

Cardiac disease	Cerebrovascular disease
Risk for heart attack	Risk for stroke
Diabetes	Arthritis
Pulmonary disorders	Visual impairments
Alcoholism	Hearing impairments
Use of sedating medications	Sleep apnea
Dementia	

TABLE 11-3. FUNCTIONAL MEASURES ASSESSED BY PRIMARY
CARE PHYSICIANS

Vision	Visuospatial skills
Hearing	Judgment
Reaction time	Muscle strength
Attention	Joint flexibility

adult drivers, when one may be dealing with multiple mild to moderate diseases (i.e., visual impairment, mild cognitive impairment, and arthritis).

Physiologic/Functional Measures
Some studies have found greater risk among physiologic variables than medical diagnoses [18]. There is a growing consensus among clinicians and experts in the field that there are many conditions and decrements in physiologic variables that can impact driving and can be easily assessed by clinicians [19–22]. The primary care physician or geriatrician can check static visual acuity [Snellen or Rosenbaum chart (see Appendix J)], hearing [whisper test (Appendix K) or hand-held audiometry], attention and reaction time (Trails A or B), visuospatial skills [Clock Completion Test (see Appendix B)], judgment, insight, muscle strength, and joint range of motion (Table 11-3). Impairments in any of these variables should be assessed for their etiologies and a treatment plan developed.

Medications
Polypharmacy is not uncommon in older adults (see Chap. 6, Approach to Polypharmacy and Appropriate Medication Use). There are many common medication classes that have been studied and noted to either increase crash risk or impair driving skills when assessed by simulators or road tests. These include but are not limited to narcotics, benzodiazepines, antihistamines, antidepressants, antipsychotics, hypnotics, medications containing alcohol, and muscle relaxants (Table 11-4) [23–25].

Health Maintenance
Clinicians should incorporate injury prevention into their health maintenance practice for older adults. Important driving issues that the clinician should discuss with the older adult driver include seat belt use, drinking alcohol, use of a cellular phone while driving, obeying the speed limit, and enrollment in refresher courses such as 55 Alive, sponsored by AARP. These are summarized in Table 11-5.

DRIVING CESSATION

There are times when the clinician may be involved in a discussion with the patient to stop driving, especially when a significant medical condition is involved. Many older

TABLE 11-4. MEDICATIONS THAT MAY IMPAIR DRIVING SKILLS

Narcotics	Antipsychotics
Benzodiazepines (agents with long half-lives appear to have higher risk than those agents with short half-lives)	Antihistamines
	Glaucoma agents
	NSAIDs
Antidepressants (agents such as tricyclics or other classes with sedating properties)	Muscle relaxants
	Medications containing alcohol
Hypnotics	

TABLE 11-5. THE PRIMARY CARE PHYSICIAN'S ROLE IN INJURY PREVENTION

Physician should reinforce the following:

Use of safety restraints

Vehicle should be in good working condition

No alcohol when driving

Obey the speed limit

Discourage use of cellular phones while driving

Review medical conditions that may impair driving skills

Consider refresher course for driving (55 Alive)

Use of safety helmets when riding motorcycles or riding bikes

---

drivers have been driving longer than their physicians have been practicing medicine. **It is important for health professionals to discuss these issues in a sensitive manner.** The physician can play an important role in enforcing driving cessation and the acceptance of the patient to stop driving their vehicle, and can suggest alternative transportation resources. These discussions should be documented in the patient's chart.

Public transportation systems [26] may have reduced fares for senior citizens. Owing to restricted sites and the physical or cognitive limitations in the older driver, these services are typically underused. State- or local- sponsored services may provide door-to-door transport for older adults in large vans, many of which are lift-equipped. Local communities, societies, retirement centers, or church groups may use funds or volunteers to provide services to physician offices, grocery stores, and meetings.

Special mention is made of the older adult driver who does not have insight into his or her own illness, such as Alzheimer's disease patients. An extensive review of the issues surrounding the driver with cognitive impairment is beyond the scope of this chapter. The interested reader is referred to a recent review on this subject [27]. The spouse or family, physician, occupational therapist, and Department of Motor Vehicles employees may need to work together to keep those individuals judged to be unsafe from driving. In situations in which the patient does not have insight, these efforts may include involving the police or Department of Revenue to confiscate the driver's license, removing access to car keys, moving the automobile off premises, changing door locks, filing down the ignition keys, or disabling the battery cable.

REFERRAL SOURCES

There are many health professionals and organizations that may assist in the education, training, or assessment of the older adult driver. These include but are not limited to subspecialists in the field of medicine (neurology, cardiology), neuropsychologists, occupational therapists, physical therapists, courses such as 55 Alive, the medical advisory board of the state or driver improvement office, and/or insurance companies. **A driving simulator is another resource to assess driving abilities,** if available to the patient and clinician.

Road performance tests are yet another method for evaluating driving skills. Road tests have some limitations. Because they are often scored subjectively, the road conditions may vary and may be performed in a car and driving course that is unfamiliar to the subject. Occupational therapists, often based at rehabilitation centers, may have specific training and experience in evaluating drivers with medical impairments. The therapist may be able to assist in modifications of the vehicle that could enable safe operation of the automobile.

The physical therapist can be an indispensable member of the driving rehabilitation team. Large studies on older adult drivers in the community indicate that back pain, arthritis [28], and the use of pain medications [29] are associated with increased crash rates. Thus, limitations in muscle strength due to pain or disuse or restrictions in range of motion of joints such as the hands, feet, and neck may play an important role in driving impairment. **Interventions to improve muscle strength and joint function have the potential to improve driving skills.**

ETHICAL, LEGAL, AND PUBLIC POLICY ISSUES

Patients and families do not always comply or agree with a clinician's recommendation to stop driving. Physicians may simply decide to document this refusal in the chart, as long as the opinion is given to someone who has decision-making capacity. However, this situation may justify a letter to the state Department of Motor Vehicles. This breach of confidentiality may be appropriate when performed in the best interest of the community [30]. The state agency will ultimately have the final decision as to whether someone can remain licensed to drive. The decision to report patients to the Department of Motor Vehicles varies depending on personal practices and state requirements. Because the common law and statutes vary among states, legal counsel should be obtained to help guide the evaluation process and determine the regulations that should apply for practices in each state. Some states, such as California, require physicians to report specific medical conditions such as dementia of the Alzheimer type.

ADDITIONAL RESOURCES

American Association for Retired Persons (AARP). Call (800) 993-7222 or visit the Web site to find out about the 55 Alive Driver Safety Program, safe driving tips, and information on aging and driving.

Area Agency on Aging (AAA). Call the Eldercare Locator number at (800) 677-1116 to connect with your local AAA. The AAA can inform you of services in your area such as ride programs, Meals-on-Wheels, home health services, and more.

Association for Driver Rehabilitation Specialists (ADED). Call ADED at (800) 290-2344 or visit the Web site to find a driver rehabilitation specialist in your area.

National Association of Social Workers (NASW). Visit the NASW Web site to locate a clinical social worker in your area. A social worker can provide counseling, assess social and emotional needs, and assist in locating and coordinating community services.

New York State Office for the Aging (NYSOFA). Visit the NYSOFA Web site to find more information and resources on helping the older driver, including *When you are concerned*, a handbook for friends, families, and caregivers concerned about the safety of an older driver.

KEY POINTS TO REMEMBER

- The ability to drive or be driven is crucial for the elderly to maintain an important link with society.
- The prevention of motor vehicle collisions should be included in the health maintenance and injury prevention program of all older adults.
- Common diseases in older adult drivers that have been noted to affect driving ability include but are not limited to visual impairment, diabetes mellitus, seizure disorders, Alzheimer's disease, cerebrovascular accidents, depression, cardiovascular disease, sleep disorders, arthritis, other related musculoskeletal disorders, and alcohol and drug use.
- Drugs that may impair driving ability and lead to increased risk of driving injuries include narcotics, benzodiazepines, antihistamines, antidepressants, antipsychotics, hypnotics, and muscle relaxants.
- Many resources are available to assist in the assessment of the older adult driver.
- Interventions to improve muscle strength and joint function have the potential to improve driving skills.
- Laws and policies regarding the physician's responsibilities to report potentially dangerous drivers vary from state to state.

SUGGESTED READING

Dobbs BM, Carr DB, Morris JC. Evaluation and management of the driver with dementia. *Neurologist* 2002;8:61–70.

Foley KT, Mitchell SJ. The elderly driver: what physicians need to know. *Cleve Clin J Med* 1997;64:423–428.

Graca JL. Driving and aging. *Clin Geriatr Med* 1986;2:577.

REFERENCES

1. Demography and epidemiology. In: Kane R, Ouslander J, Abrass I, eds. *Essentials of clinical geriatrics*. New York: McGraw-Hill, 1984:21.
2. Rice D, MacKenzie E. *Cost of injury in the United States: a report to congress*. San Francisco, CA: Institute for Health and Aging, University of California and Injury Prevention Center, The Johns Hopkins University, 1989.
3. Evans L. Older driver involvement in fatal and severe traffic crashes. *J Gerontol* 1988;43:S189.
4. Marottoli RA, Richardson ED, Stowe MH, et al. Development of a test battery to identify older drivers at risk for self-reported adverse driving events. *J Am Geriatr Soc* 1998;46:562–568.
5. Sabey BE, Staughton GC. *Interacting roles of road environment, vehicle and road use in accidents*. London: 5th International Conference of the International Association of Accident and Traffic Medicine, 1975.
6. Koepsell TD, Wolf ME, McCloskey L, et al. Medical conditions and motor vehicle collision injuries in older adults. *J Am Geriatr Soc* 1994;42:695–700.
7. Gallo JJ, Rebok GW, Lesikar SE. The driving habits of adults aged 60 years and older. *J Am Geriatr Soc* 1999;47:335–341.
8. Shinar D, Schieber F. Visual requirements for safety and mobility of older drivers. *Hum Factors* 1991;33:505–519.
9. Crancer JA Jr, McMurray L. Accident and violation rates of Washington's medically restricted drivers. *JAMA* 1968;205:272–276.
10. Hansotia P, Broste SK. The effect of epilepsy or diabetes mellitus on the risk of automobile accidents. *N Engl J Med* 1991;324:22–26.
11. Drachman DA, Swearer JM. Driving and Alzheimer's disease: the risk of crashes. *Neurology* 1993;42:2448–2456.
12. Wilson T, Smith T. Driving after stroke. *Int Rehabil Med* 1983;5:170–177.
13. Doege TC, Engelberg AL, eds. *Medical conditions affecting drivers*. Chicago: American Medical Association, 1986.
14. Waller JA. Chronic medical conditions and traffic safety: review of the California experience. *N Engl J Med* 1965;273:1413–1420.
15. Findley LJ, Unverzagt ME, Suratt PM. Automobile accidents involving patients with obstructive sleep apnea. *Am Rev Respir Dis* 1988;138:337–340.
16. Roberts WN, Roberts P. Evaluation of the elderly driver with arthritis. *Clin Geriatr Med* 1993;9:311–322.
17. Ray WA, Gurwitz J, Decker MD, et al. Medications and the safety of the older driver: is there a basis for concern? *Hum Factors* 1992;34(1):33–47.
18. Sims RV, Owsley C, Allman RM, et al. A preliminary assessment of the medical and functional factors associated with vehicle crashes by older adults. *J Am Geriatr Soc* 1998;46:556–561.
19. Reuben D. Assessment of older drivers. *Clin Geriatr Med* 1993;9:449–459.
20. Underwood M. The older driver. Clinical assessment and injury prevention. *Arch Intern Med* 1992;152:735–740.
21. Foley KT, Mitchell SJ. The elderly driver: what physicians need to know. *Cleve Clin J Med* 1997;64:423–428.
22. Marottoli RA, Cooney LM, Wagener DR, et al. Predictors of automobile crashes and moving violations among elderly drivers. *Ann Intern Med* 1994;121:842–846.
23. Hemmelgarn B, Suissa S, Huang A, et al. Benzodiazepine use and the risk of motor vehicle crash in the elderly. *JAMA* 1997;278:27–31.

24. Higgins JP, Wright SW, Wrenn KD. Alcohol, the elderly, and motor vehicle crashes. *Am J Emerg Med* 1996;14:265–267.
25. Johansson K, Bryding G, Dahl ML, et al. Traffic dangerous drugs are often found in fatally injured older male drivers. *J Am Geriatr Soc* 1997;45:1029–1031.
26. Roper TA, Mulley GP. Caring for older people. Public transport. *BMJ* 1996;313: 415–418.
27. Dobbs BM, Carr DB, Morris JC. Evaluation and management of the driver with dementia. *Neurologist* 2002;8:61–70.
28. Foley DJ, Wallace RB, Eberhard J. Risk factors for motor vehicle crashes among older drivers in a rural community. *J Am Geriatr Soc* 1995;43:776–781.
29. Tuokko H, Beattie BC, Tallman K, et al. Predictors of motor vehicle crashes in a dementia clinic population: the role of gender and arthritis. *J Am Geriatr Soc* 1995;43:1444–1445.
30. Graca JL. Driving and aging. *Clin Geriatr Med* 1986;2:577.

12

Androgen Deficiency in Older Men

Kyle C. Moylan

INTRODUCTION

Epidemiology

Androgen deficiency is common in the male geriatric population. Testosterone levels begin to decrease in the fifth decade of life and continue to decline with age. The prevalence of free or bioavailable testosterone levels considered deficient in comparison to young controls is approximately 10% in the sixth decade and 70% in the eighth decade of life [1]. Although this occurrence is sometimes referred to as the **andropause**, it differs from female menopause in many ways. Unlike menopause, not all men are affected, and the decline in gonadal function is more gradual.

CAUSES

Pathophysiology

Testosterone is the most important androgen in men. Testosterone is produced and secreted by Leydig cells of the testes under the control of leuteinizing hormone (LH) and gonadotropin-releasing hormone. Testosterone is converted in target tissues to its more active form, dihydroxytestosterone, by 5-alpha reductase.

The decline in testosterone with advancing age may be due to central (hypothalamic-pituitary) and peripheral (testicular) alterations. There is an age-related decrease in the size and weight of the testes as well as a decline in the number and volume of the Leydig cells. The normal diurnal variation in the secretion of testosterone is also blunted or lost with age. In addition, many men do not exhibit an appropriate increase in levels of LH, an indicator of hypothalamic-pituitary dysfunction [2]. Finally, **testosterone is highly protein-bound, predominately to sex-hormone–binding globulin.** Sex-hormone–binding globulin levels increase with age, resulting in a decrease in free or bioavailable testosterone.

The gradual decline in androgens that accompanies normal aging can be worsened by comorbid conditions. Several medical conditions and drugs are known to result in androgen deficiency (Tables 12-1 and 12-2).

PRESENTATION

Clinical Features

The clinical features of androgen deficiency are many and nonspecific, frequently overlapping with the features of other geriatric syndromes or unsuccessful aging. **Low testosterone has been associated with decreased libido, depressive symptoms, erectile dysfunction, cognitive impairment, anemia, and loss of secondary sexual characteristics.** Androgen deficiency may be a risk factor for dementia.

Important changes in body composition include loss of muscle and bone mass. Sarcopenia and decreased muscle strength may develop. **Androgen deficiency is a known cause of osteoporosis and a risk factor for osteoporotic fractures.** Abdomi-

TABLE 12-1. CONDITIONS ASSOCIATED WITH ANDROGEN DEFICIENCY

Cirrhosis	Chronic infections or inflammation
Chronic renal failure	Debilitation
Hemochromatosis	Thalassemia
Amyloidosis	Surgical castration
Zinc deficiency	Sickle cell anemia
Orchitis	HIV
COPD	Medications (see Table 12-2)
Rheumatoid arthritis	

nal fat increases, and there may be an increase in insulin resistance. The reported effect on lipids has been mixed.

History

As previously mentioned, many of the symptoms of androgen deficiency are nonspecific. **Patients should be questioned regarding mood, erectile function, libido, hair loss (changes in shaving), fractures, weakness, and fatigue.** Screening tools are available to systematically investigate the presence of symptoms (see Appendix G), with reasonable sensitivity and specificity [3].

Historical features that may indicate a cause of androgen deficiency should be sought, including vision changes (pituitary adenomas), head trauma, testicular trauma or infection (mumps orchitis), liver disease, and medications (especially for prostate cancer; Table 12-2).

Other symptoms to inquire about may guide therapy, such as a history or symptoms of prostate disease, sleep apnea, or polycythemia.

TABLE 12-2. MEDICATIONS THAT AFFECT TESTOSTERONE FUNCTION

Medications that decrease testosterone levels
  Gonadotropin-releasing hormone agonist or antagonists [leuprolide (Lupron)]
  Glucocorticoids
  Ketoconazole
  Spironolactone
  Thiazides
  Opiates
  Amiodarone
  Psychotropics
  Anabolic steroids
  Estrogens
  Progestins
Medications that impair testosterone at the receptor
  Cimetidine
  Flutamide
  Spironolactone
  Androgen antagonists

Physical Exam

The physical exam should focus on **body hair distribution, breast size, genitalia, musculature, strength, visual fields, and the prostate.** Functional assessment helps determine the possible impact of androgen deficiency on routine activities.

Diagnostic Evaluation

Signs and symptoms consistent with androgen deficiency should initially be evaluated with a **total testosterone level, preferably drawn in the morning.** Normal values in healthy young adults range from 300–1000 ng/dL. A level <300 ng/dL confirms the diagnosis. If signs and symptoms are present but the total testosterone is normal, a more sensitive test, either a free or bioavailable testosterone, is indicated.

A lab diagnosis of androgen deficiency should be followed up with the measurement of prolactin, TSH, and LH. An elevated prolactin or low LH is an indication for an MRI of the sella and hypothalamus. **Bone densitometry should be considered at the time of diagnosis.**

MANAGEMENT

Treatment

The clinical features of androgen deficiency have been effectively treated with testosterone replacement in young patients. Little is known, however, about the long-term efficacy and safety of testosterone therapy in older hypogonadal men. The decision to start testosterone therapy needs to be individualized, with the hope of improving specific outcomes weighed against potential adverse effects. Comorbid conditions that could also explain the same symptoms (depression) should be treated.

Several small short-term (<3 yrs) studies have demonstrated improvements of various aspects of androgen deficiency in the elderly. **These include increased lean body weight, decreased abdominal fat, improved grip strength, increased bone mineral density, increased libido, and improved cognitive function** [4,5]. Data are lacking for the impact on quality of life, functional measures, mood, and cardiovascular events.

Potential adverse effects of testosterone replacement include worsening obstructive sleep apnea, acne, gynecomastia, testicular atrophy, aggression, and polycythemia. Testosterone probably does not increase the risk of prostate cancer but may exacerbate existing disease. It is not clear if treatment contributes to or worsens benign prostatic hyperplasia. The effects of testosterone therapy on lipids have been mixed, although there appears to be no impact on inflammatory markers [6,7].

Contraindications to testosterone replacement are a diagnosis or history of breast cancer, prostate cancer, polycythemia, untreated obstructive sleep apnea, drug sensitivity, or moderate to severe obstructive symptoms of benign prostatic hyperplasia.

Several forms of testosterone are available for use in the United States: IM injection, scrotal patch, nonscrotal patch, and topical gel. Each method has advantages and disadvantages (Table 12-3). **The specific route of testosterone administration needs to be customized to the patient's needs.** Factors that need to be considered include convenience, ability or willingness to administer therapy (use the gel correctly or shave the scrotum), and cost.

Follow-Up

If the decision is made to initiate treatment with testosterone, the patient's clinical response and tolerance should be closely monitored. Before initiating treatment, check the baseline prostate-specific antigen, lipids, Hct, and digital rectal exam. At 3 mos, these studies should be repeated and followed at least annually thereafter [8]. Clinical improvement in symptoms of androgen deficiency usually begins within 1 mo. Lack of a clinical response may indicate treatment failure, inadequate dosage (consider checking levels), or an alternative diagnosis as the cause of the patient's symptoms.

TABLE 12-3. TESTOSTERONE REPLACEMENT THERAPIES

Treatment	Route	Dosage	Advantages	Disadvantages
Testosterone enanthate Testosterone cypionate	IM	150–200 mg q2–3wks	Infrequent dosing Least expensive	Fluctuating serum levels—supra-physiologic levels after the first few days followed by subphysiologic levels before the next dose
				More difficult to monitor and interpret serum levels
				May require an office visit for some patients
				Injection site pain
Testoderm	Scrotal patch applied daily	4–6 mg/day	More physiologic testosterone levels than injections	Requires shaving scrotum
				Must keep area dry
				Local irritation
			Easier to assess serum levels	More expensive than injections
Testoderm TTS	Patch applied daily to nonscrotal, non-hair–bearing skin	5 mg/day	More physio-logic testoster-one levels than injec-tions	Local irritation, con-tact dermatitis
				More expensive than injections
			Easier to assess serum levels	
Androderm	Patch changed daily to nonscrotal, non-hair–bearing skin	5–10 mg/day	More physiologic testosterone levels than injections	Local irritation, con-tact dermatitis
				More expensive than injections
			Easier to assess serum levels	
Testosterone gel (Andro-Gel)	Topical gel	5–10 g/day	More physiologic testosterone levels than injections	Limited ability to titrate dose
				Area must be kept dry up to 6 hrs after application
			Easy to apply	Can transfer testos-terone to others through skin con-tact
				Most expensive route

KEY POINTS TO REMEMBER

- Androgen deficiency is common in older men due to a gradual decline in testosterone production with age.
- Numerous medical conditions and medications are associated with male androgen deficiency.
- Potential clinical consequences of androgen deficiency include sexual dysfunction, depressive symptoms, cognitive impairment, dementia, anemia, sarcopenia, osteoporosis, and functional decline.
- Suspected androgen deficiency can be confirmed by measurement of a decreased total testosterone level. In some instances, the total testosterone level is in the low-normal range, and measurement of the free or bioavailable testosterone is required to establish the diagnosis.
- Limited data are available regarding the efficacy and safety of long-term testosterone therapy.
- Multiple formulations of testosterone are available to meet individual patient needs, including injections, topical patches, and topical gels.

REFERENCES

1. Harman SM, Metter EJ, Tobin JD, et al. Longitudinal effects of aging on serum total and free testosterone levels in healthy men. Baltimore Longitudinal Study of Aging. *J Clin Endocrinol Metab* 2001;86:724–731.
2. Morley JE, Kaiser FE, Perry HM 3rd, et al. Longitudinal changes in testosterone, luteinizing hormone, and follicle-stimulating hormone in healthy older men. *Metabolism* 1997;46:410–413.
3. Morley JE, Charlton E, Patrick P, et al. Validation of a screening questionnaire for androgen deficiency in aging males. *Metabolism* 2000;49:1239–1242.
4. Cherrier MM, Asthana S, Plymate S, et al. Testosterone supplementation improves spatial and verbal memory in healthy older men. *Neurology* 2001;57: 80–88.
5. Basaria S, Dobs AS. Hypogonadism and androgen replacement therapy in elderly men. *Am J Med* 2001;110:563–572.
6. Snyder PJ, Peachey H, Berlin JA, et al. Effect of transdermal testosterone treatment on lipids and apolipoproteins in men over 65. *Am J Med* 2001;11:255–260.
7. Ng MK, Liu PY, Williams AJ, et al. Prospective study of effect of androgens of serum inflammatory markers in men. *Arterioscler Thromb Vasc Biol* 2002;22: 1136–1141.
8. Cunningham GR, Swerdloff RS, et al. Summary from the Second Annual Andropause Consensus Meeting. The Endocrine Society, 2001.

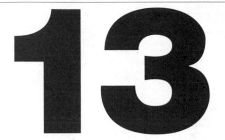

Sex Hormone Therapy in the Elderly Woman

Stanley J. Birge

INTRODUCTION

Sex hormone therapy (HT) in the elderly woman is controversial because of the potential increased risks of adverse outcomes. These risks and benefits depend on the type of HT, the age of the patient, and other patient-related factors. **Therefore, each patient must be evaluated for the risks and benefits of HT.**

PHYSIOLOGY

Menopause is a consequence of a decline in ovarian production of estradiol that occurs during the fifth to sixth decade of life or at any earlier age because of surgical or pharmacologic intervention. The immediate consequence of ovarian failure is highly variable with respect to vasomotor symptoms, changes in mood, memory, concentration, and sleep disturbance, with many patients being asymptomatic. Surgical menopause may also be associated with symptoms of testosterone deficiency. The intermediate and long-term consequences of estrogen deficiency are the focus of this chapter (Table 13-1).

ADVERSE EFFECTS OF HORMONE THERAPY

Venous Thromboembolic Disease

The risk of pulmonary embolism and deep vein thrombosis combined approaches 50/10,000 patients treated in the first year, subsequently declining over the next 5 yrs to near baseline rates [1]. These data suggest that there is a vulnerable population at risk. **A previous history of spontaneous venous thrombotic disease on HT should be considered a relative contraindication for HT initiation.**

Coronary Heart Disease

During the first year of therapy with estrogen combined with the progestin, medroxyprogesterone acetate (MPA), there is an excess incidence of approximately 20 clinical and subclinical cases of coronary artery disease (CAD) events per 10,000 patients treated [1]. This rate drops to baseline by the second year. This excess incidence of cardiovascular events is not seen in observational studies in which women are initiated on HT primarily at the time of the menopause. The differences between clinical trial and observational studies have been attributed to the healthy user bias affecting observational studies or to preexisting CAD in the clinical trials in which HT was initiated after menopause at an average age of $\geq$ 63 yrs. Statin use appears to eliminate the excess incidence of coronary artery events associated with HT [2,3].

Stroke

Combined estrogen + MPA is associated with an excess of 8 strokes per 10,000 patients treated per year [1]. This excess incidence becomes evident after the first year and returns to baseline after the fourth or fifth year.

TABLE 13-1. CONSEQUENCES OF THE ESTROGEN DEFICIENCY STATE

Intermediate consequences

Redistribution of body fat from peripheral to central sites

Accelerated aging of the skin

Impaired wound healing

Increased expression of proinflammatory cytokines resulting in accelerated bone loss

Increased requirement for vitamin D to maintain bone mineral homeostasis

Urogenital atrophy

Long-term consequences

Osteoporosis

Tooth loss

Hip fracture

Acceleration of cardiovascular disease

Increased expression of colon cancer

Accelerated decline in cognitive function

Accelerated expression of Alzheimer's disease

Expression of more malignant forms of breast cancer

Cataract formation

Macular degeneration

Breast Cancer

HT is associated with an excess incidence of invasive breast cancer. The Women's Health Initiative study of estrogen + MPA does not provide a reliable estimate of that incidence, because the duration of the study averaged only 5.2 yrs, and the excess events were seen in only those few women who were using HT before the initiation of the study. Thus, it is necessary to rely on observational studies that suggest the incidence of invasive breast cancer increases after 5 yrs of use to 60 excess cases per 10,000 women treated for 10 yrs [4]. These data represent an underestimate of the true excess incidence, because few of the women were taking a progestin. Observational studies suggest that addition of a progestin to HT increases the risk of breast cancer over that of estrogen alone, with the greatest risk associated with testosterone-derived progestins. **Although unopposed estrogen is also associated with an increased incidence of breast cancer, the resulting breast cancer has a better prognosis.** Breast cancer diagnosed after ≥ 5 yrs of HT has a 50% reduced mortality compared to breast cancer in non-HT users. This reduction in mortality is seen even in those studies in which the control group had the same mammography surveillance as the estrogen-treated women.

Dementia

Initiation of HT after age 60 yrs is associated with a twofold increased risk of dementia. As with CAD, this increase may be limited to a vulnerable subgroup of women.

Endometrial Cancer

Unopposed estrogen therapy results in an increased incidence of endometrial hyperplasia and endometrial cancer but not an increased mortality from endometrial cancer. This increased incidence can be eliminated by the addition of progestin to the regimen. **Because the stimulatory effect of estrogen on the endometrium is dose dependent, the dose and frequency of progestin cycling required to prevent endometrial hyperplasia is also dependent on the estrogen dose.**

RECOMMENDATIONS FOR THE MANAGEMENT OF THE POSTMENOPAUSAL WOMAN

At the time of the menopause, a discussion of the risks and benefits of HT should be initiated by the physician with all women with or without menopausal symptoms. In women who have elected to initiate HT for menopausal symptoms, that discussion should be repeated at frequent intervals to ascertain whether to continue or modify her HT (Table 13-2). That discussion should include an assessment of the patient's risks for osteoporosis, cardiovascular disease, colon cancer, and Alzheimer's disease (AD) and her concerns for the adverse effects of HT. These discussions should also include the increasing evidence that the prevention of the long-term consequences of estrogen deficiency, specifically AD, cardiovascular disease, age-related cognitive decline, and osteoporosis, requires the initiation of HT at the time of the menopause. **For example, initiation of HT before age 65 yrs is associated with up to an 83% reduction in the incidence of AD, whereas initiation after age 60 yrs was associated with a twofold increase of dementia** [5]. These results have been confirmed by the Women's Health Initiative Memory Study, a randomized clinical trial [6]. This trial and other ongoing trials do not address the effect of initiating HT at the time of menopause. For every 1000 women treated for 10 yrs beginning at the time of the menopause, the lifetime risk of developing AD will be reduced by 240 cases at a cost of six additional cases of invasive breast cancer [7]. This evidence, although based on observational data, is sufficiently compelling to share with our patients. Furthermore, because the outcomes of AD and CAD occur some 15–30 yrs after initiation of the intervention, these associations will never be confirmed by clinical trials.

The form of HT initiated at the time of the menopause is beyond the scope of this chapter. There seems to be a consensus that **estrogen combined with daily or monthly cycling with a progestin should not be initiated or continued for the prevention of the long-term consequences of estrogen deficiency. This may not be the case for the woman on unopposed estrogen.** For the woman with a uterus, in whom the continuation of estrogen is desired, the goal is to reduce exposure to the progestin. If she has been on the combination for 3–5 yrs, she is no longer at increased risk of a cardiovascular event. However, continuation of daily or monthly cycling with a progestin increases her risk of breast cancer. **Reduction of exposure to the progestin can be accomplished by reducing gradually the dose of estrogen to the equivalent of 0.3 mg of conjugated estrogens (CEs) and then cycling q6mos or longer with progesterone or a progesterone-derived progestin for 2 wks.** In the woman without a uterus, 0.3 mg of CE may also be advantageous with respect to breast tenderness and breast cancer risk. However, in the woman concerned about osteoporosis, dual-energy x-ray absorptiometry bone densitometry is indicated to determine whether this dose is sufficient to maintain skeletal integrity. The efficacy and safety of low-dose regimens have not been adequately studied.

TABLE 13-2. INDICATIONS FOR CONTINUATION OF HORMONE THERAPY

Family history of Alzheimer's disease	Quality-of-life issues
Family history of heart disease	Sleep quality
Family history of osteoporosis	Enjoyment of sexual activity
	Cognitive function
	Mood

DURATION OF HORMONAL THERAPY

The benefits of HT for mental health and AD appear to be achieved primarily in the first 10–15 yrs of use. There is insufficient data to indicate that use beyond this period would be of benefit except for the prevention of hip fracture and colon cancer. It should be noted that bisphosphonates are not effective in the prevention of hip fracture in women over age 80 yrs when 75% of hip fractures occur [8] (see Chap. 14, Osteoporosis). Thus, until we better understand causes of hip fracture, continuation of HT may be a prudent alternative in those at increased risk. Because longevity and quality of life are improved with HT, continuation of low-dose HT (0.3 mg CE) is justified. The increased risk of breast and uterine cancer may be offset by the associated decrease in mortality from these cancers and colon cancer.

WHEN TO INITIATE HORMONE THERAPY

Prevention of CAD, AD, and age-related cognitive decline appear to require the initiation of HT early, if not at the time of the menopause, for maximum benefit. Initiation of HT after the menopause transition is associated with an increased risk of stroke, dementia, and CAD. HT should not be initiated in the older adult for the treatment or prevention of these disorders. Using the lowest effective dose of estrogen and limiting exposure to progestins can reduce the risks of adverse events (Table 13-3).

TABLE 13-3. COMMON DRUGS FOR HORMONE THERAPY

Preparation	Daily maintenance dose	Formulations
Conjugated equine estrogens	0.3–0.625 mg PO	0.3, 0.625, 0.9, 1.25, 2.5 mg PO
Premarin		
Conjugated synthetic estrogens	0.3–0.625 mg PO	0.3, 0.625, 0.9 mg PO
Cenestin		
Estropipate	0.625–1.25 mg PO	0.625, 1.25, 2.5 mg PO
Ogen		
Esterified estrogen	0.3–0.625 mg PO	0.3, 0.625, 1.25, 2.5 mg PO
Estratab, Menest		
Micronized 17β-estradiol	0.5–1 mg PO	0.5, 1, 2 mg PO
Estrace		
Transdermal estrogen	0.025–0.075 mg/day	
Alora		0.05, 0.075, 0.1 mg/day biweekly
Estraderm		0.05, 0.1 mg/day biweekly
Vivelle		0.0375, 0.05, 0.075, 0.1 mg/day biweekly
Climara		0.05, 0.075, 0.1 mg/day weekly
FemPatch		0.025 mg/day weekly
Progesterone	100–200 mg PO × 10–14 days	100, 200 mg PO
Prometrium		
Medroxyprogesterone	2.5–10 mg PO × 10–14 days	2.5, 5, 10 mg PO
Provera, Cycrin		

KEY POINTS TO REMEMBER

- HT may dramatically improve the quality of life for some menopausal women and prevents or delays the expression of cardiovascular and neurodegenerative diseases that represent the major causes of disability and the loss of independence in the older adult woman.
- To maximize these benefits, HT should be initiated early and continued for at least 10–15 yrs.
- Effects on hip fracture, colon cancer, and quality-of-life issues probably require continued use of HT.
- The adverse effects of HT are dependent on the dose of estrogen and the addition of a progestin.
- Estrogen combined with daily or monthly cycling with a progestin should not be initiated or continued for the prevention of the long-term consequences of the estrogen deficiency state.
- The increased incidence of breast and uterine cancer associated with HT appears to be offset by the decrease in mortality from these cancers and colon cancer.

REFERENCES

1. Writing Group for the Women's Health Initiative Investigators. Risk and benefits of estrogen plus progestin in healthy postmenopausal women; principal results from the women's Health Initiative randomized controlled trial. *JAMA* 2002;288:321–333
2. Mendelsohn ME, Karas RH. The time has come to stop letting the HERS tale wag the dogma. *Circulation* 2001;104:2256–2257.
3. Herrington DM, Vittinghoff E, Lin F, et al. Statin therapy, cardiovascular events, and total mortality in the Heart and Estrogen/progestin Replacement Study (HERS). *Circulation* 2002;105:2962–2967.
4. Collaborative Group on Hormonal Factors in Breast Cancer. Breast cancer and hormone replacement therapy: collaborative reanalysis of data from 51 epidemiological studies of 52,705 women with breast cancer and 108,411 women without breast cancer. *Lancet* 1997;350:1047–1059.
5. Zandi PP, Carlson MC, Plassman BL, et al. Hormone replacement therapy and incidence of Alzheimer's disease in older women. The Cache County Study. *JAMA* 2002;288:2123–2129.
6. Shumaker SA, Legault C, Rapp SR, et al. Estrogen plus progestin and the incidence of dementia and mild cognitive impairment in postmenopausal women: the Women's Health Initiative Memory Study: a randomized controlled trial. *JAMA* 2003;289:2651–2662.
7. Birge SJ. The use of estrogen in older women. *Clin Geriatr Med* 2003;19:617–627.
8. McClung MR, Geusens P, Miller PD, et al. Effect of risedronate on the risk of hip fracture in elderly women. *N Engl J Med* 2001;344:333–340.

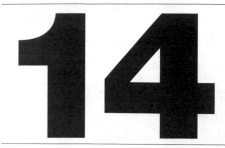

Osteoporosis

Divya Shroff and
Latha Sivaprasad

INTRODUCTION

Osteoporosis is one of the most common ailments affecting the geriatric population, and it is not a concern for women alone. Osteoporosis affects an estimated 10 million people, and an additional 18 million have low bone mass. 25 million American women and 1.5 million American men (age group $\geq$ 65 yrs) are affected by osteoporosis. Osteoporosis is an asymptomatic disease that needs to be **screened for and treated before the first fracture occurs.** After a hip fracture, almost one-third of geriatric patients are discharged to a nursing home.

Osteoporosis as defined by the WHO is bone mineral density (BMD) that is at least 2.5 SDs below the standard mean for young adults of the same sex (T-score of $\leq$–2.5). A T-score between –1 and –2.5 defines **osteopenia** (Tables 14-1 and 14-2).

CAUSES

Pathogenesis

Bone density and bone quality both contribute to bone strength. Osteoporosis results from the uncoupling of bone resorption (osteoclastic activity) and bone formation (osteoblastic activity). Table 14-3 lists the causes of osteoporosis.

PRESENTATION

Diagnostic Evaluation

It is important to remember that osteoporosis is an **asymptomatic** metabolic disorder. Therefore, it is essential to screen all appropriate patients and start therapy before the first fracture occurs (Table 14-4).

Assessing Bone Mass

DUAL-ENERGY X-RAY ABSORPTIOMETRY. In **dual-energy x-ray absorptiometry** (DEXA), two energy beams are passed through bone (usually of the hip and spine) and compared to a standardized control. This results in a **T-score,** which is the number of SDs above or below the mean BMD for gender and race matched to young controls. BMD at the hip correlates best with the risk of hip fracture, and BMD at the spine correlates best with the risk of vertebral fractures.

QUANTITATIVE U/S. **Quantitative U/S** of the heel has been studied and is an inexpensive screen for osteoporosis. **DEXA scanning should be used to confirm diagnosis and monitor treatment.**

Assessing Bone Metabolism

Assessing bone metabolism through biochemical markers reflects more acute changes in bone remodeling compared to DEXA scanning, but they do not predict bone mass or fracture risk. They are of limited value in following response to therapy:

- **Bone formation:** alkaline phosphatase, osteocalcin, procollagen I carboxy peptide
- **Bone resorption:** hydroxyproline, N-telopeptide, collagen cross-link molecules

TABLE 14-1. T-SCORE DIAGNOSIS

≤ –2.5	Osteoporosis
Between –1 and –2.5	Osteopenia
≥ –1	Normal

SECONDARY CAUSES

Secondary causes should be excluded by measuring CBC, BUN, creatinine, **serum calcium, TSH,** liver function tests, **25-hydroxy vitamin D, testosterone level (in men), and 24-hr urine collection for calcium and creatinine.** Serum protein electrophoresis and intact PTH may also be appropriate.

MANAGEMENT

Treatment

The goal of treatment is to reduce the incidence of bone fractures. The decision to treat should be individualized based on the patient's willingness to accept treatment (for a silent disease), risk of fracture, and comorbidities.

Nonspecific Management for All Patients, Regardless of Bone Mineral Density
The diagnosis of osteoporosis should trigger an assessment of fall risk (see Chap. 7, Falls) with the appropriate interventions.

All patients should be advised to maintain physical activity. Resistance training can improve BMD, but other forms of exercise are beneficial by reducing the risk of falls.

Secondary causes of osteoporosis should be treated.

Adequate calcium and vitamin D intake should be advised for all patients:

* **Calcium** intake should be 1000–1500 mg PO qd, which may require calcium supplements.
  * Dosing: calcium carbonate (Tums 200/300/400 mg) taken in divided doses.
  * Concerns: monitor for constipation and other GI side effects.
* **Vitamin D, 400–800 IU/day,** is recommended for patients >65 yrs to promote intestinal absorption of calcium. The dose needs to be increased if the 24-hr urine calcium/creatinine ratio is <0.15. Pharmacologic doses of vitamin D (50,000 U monthly or weekly) may be required for patients with deficiency or resistance to vitamin D. Dosing is monitored by the 24-hr urinary calcium and creatinine.

Specific Pharmacologic Treatment
Specific pharmacologic treatment should be offered to

* All patients with a T-score of ≤ –2 in the absence of risk factors for fracture
* Patients with a T-score of –1.5 to –2 with one or more risk factors besides menopause
* Anyone with a fracture suspected to be secondary to osteoporosis

TABLE 14-2. PREDICTORS OF BONE MASS

Predictors of low bone mass

Female gender, increased age, white or Asian race, low estrogen states, low weight and BMI, low calcium intake, positive family history, history of falls or fractures, smoking, inactivity, >1.5-in. loss of height

Predictors of high bone mass

Regular exercise, good nutrition, normal puberty

TABLE 14-3.   CAUSES OF OSTEOPOROSIS

Primary osteoporosis	Postmenopausal
	Idiopathic
	Juvenile osteoporosis
Secondary osteoporosis	Steroids and Cushing's syndrome
	Hypogonadism
	Hyperthyroidism
	Diabetes mellitus
	Anorexia nervosa
	Hyperparathyroidism
	Malabsorption (celiac disease, cystic fibrosis, irritable bowel disease)
	Medications (steroids, anticonvulsants)
	Toxins (smoking)
	Liver disease
	Renal disease
	Malnutrition (low vitamin D and calcium intake)
	Multiple myeloma
	Rheumatoid arthritis
	Sarcoidosis

BISPHOSPHONATES.   **Bisphosphonates are the most effective drugs for reducing the risk of vertebral and nonvertebral fractures in patients with osteoporosis.** The effects on BMD are comparable to those of hormone therapy (HT). Bisphosphonates act by inhibiting osteoclastic bone resorption.

Dosing.   Second-generation drugs are more effective and have been shown to reduce the risk of vertebral and nonvertebral fractures, including hip fractures, in women <80 yrs [1,2]:

- **Alendronate: 70 mg PO every week** [3].
- **Risedronate: 35 mg PO every week.**
- Zoledronic acid (IV) has been shown to improve BMD [4], but fracture data are not available to date. It has an extremely long duration of action and may allow for treatment annually. It is currently not FDA approved for the treatment of osteoporosis.

Concerns.   Esophageal irritation and ulceration and occasional myalgias and arthralgias are potential adverse effects. **Bisphosphonates have poor intestinal**

TABLE 14-4.   INDICATIONS TO ASSESS BONE MASS

Postmenopausal women willing to undergo treatment

Age >65 yrs

History of osteoporotic fracture

Steroid use for ≥ 2 mos

Risk factors for osteoporosis (see Tables 14-2 and 14-3)

Monitoring therapy

absorption and low bioavailability. The patient must take the medication on an empty stomach with a full glass of water, then remain upright without food intake for at least 30 mins. Avoid use in patients with upper GI diseases, gastroesophageal reflux disease, and achalasia.

ESTROGEN. Estrogen should be considered for female patients (see Chap. 13, Sex Hormone Therapy in the Elderly Woman). BMD correlates strongly with lifetime estrogen exposure. To prevent the 20% loss of BMD at the time of menopause, HT should be initiated earlier and continued. In contrast to bisphosphonates, HT prevents osteoporotic nonvertebral fractures in women older than 80 yrs and in women without osteoporosis (T-score <−2.5). HT is an established approach to the treatment and prevention of osteoporosis. Observational and prospective studies have shown a fracture reduction of 35–50%.

Dosing. See Chap. 13, Sex Hormone Therapy in the Elderly Woman.

Concerns. HT remains controversial. The decision to begin HT should be based on patient and physician preference after considering the possible benefits and risks. The possible risks include higher incidence of breast cancer, stroke, venous thromboembolism, cholelithiasis, and uterine bleeding.

The combination of HT and bisphosphonates marginally exceeds the benefits of either separately and is not recommended.

SELECTIVE ESTROGEN RECEPTOR MODULATORS. Selective estrogen receptor modulators have a limited role in the treatment of osteoporosis. These are designed to have mixed agonist and antagonist effects on estrogen receptors. This results in a protective bone effect and up to a 50% decreased risk of breast cancer within 3–5 yrs of use. Increased BMD and decrease in vertebral fractures has been demonstrated [5]. Raloxifene has not been shown to decrease the risk of nonvertebral fractures. Unlike tamoxifen, raloxifene may not increase the risk of developing endometrial cancer.

Dosing. Raloxifene, 60 mg PO daily.

Concerns. The patient may have increased risk of venous thromboembolism. Risk of invasive breast cancer may increase after 5 yrs as seen with tamoxifen.

CALCITONIN. Calcitonin also has a limited role in the treatment of osteoporosis. This agent inhibits osteoclastic bone resorption and decreases bone pain. Studies have shown a 1–2% increase in BMD and decreased incidence of vertebral fracture but no effect on nonvertebral or hip fractures.

Dosing. Intranasal spray is 200 IU per day.

Concerns. Patients have shown the ability to form resistance, and once discontinued, the benefits are transient.

Follow-Up

Currently, there are no consensus recommendations to monitor treatment efficacy and compliance. A repeated DEXA scan up to 2 yrs after initiating treatment can be useful in reevaluating the impact of therapy on BMD. After 1 yr, there may be loss of BMD, but with continued treatment, BMD may still increase.

KEY POINTS TO REMEMBER

- Osteoporosis is an asymptomatic disease that needs to be screened for by primary care physicians and geriatricians.
- Osteoporosis can be primary or secondary to other conditions.
- Indications to measure bone density include postmenopausal women willing to undergo treatment, history of osteoporotic fracture, presence of risk factors for osteoporosis, or monitoring treatment.
- BMD of the hip by DEXA measurement is the best predictor of hip fracture.
- The T-score is used to define osteoporosis (T-score of <−2.5) and osteopenia (T-score between −1 and −2.5).
- All patients with low bone density should be evaluated for fall risk and be advised to maintain physical activity along with adequate intake of calcium and vitamin D.
- Effective medications are available for the reduction of osteoporotic fracture risk.

SUGGESTED READING

Eastell R. Treatment of postmenopausal osteoporosis. *N Engl J Med* 1998;338:736–745.

McGarry KA, Kiel DP. Postmenopausal osteoporosis. *Postgrad Med* 2000;108:79–91.

McClung MR, Geusens P, Miller PD, et al. Effect of risedronate on the risk of hip fracture in elderly women. *N Engl J Med* 2001;344:333–340.

The MORE Investigators. Reduction of vertebral fracture risk in postmenopausal women with osteoporosis treated with raloxifene. *JAMA* 1999;282:637–645.

Orwoll E, Ettinger M, Weiss S, et al. Alendronate for the treatment of osteoporosis in men. *N Engl J Med* 2000;343(9):604–610.

Osteoporosis prevention, diagnosis, and therapy. *NIH Consensus Statement* 2000;17 (1):1–36.

Reid IR, Brown JP, Burckhardt P, et al. Intravenous zoledronic acid in postmenopausal women with low bone mineral density. *N Engl J Med* 2002;346:653–661.

Schnitzer T, Bone HG, Crepaldi G, et al. Therapeutic equivalence of alendronate 70 mg once weekly and alendronate 10mg daily in the treatment of osteoporosis. *Aging Clin Exp Res* 2000;12(1):1–12.

Siddiqui NA, Shetty KR, Duthie EH Jr. Osteoporosis in older men: discovering when and how to treat it. *Geriatrics* 1999;54:20–28.

Simonelli C. Pharmaceutical approaches to managing osteoporosis in postmenopausal women. *Nursing Home Med* 1997;5:H1–H8.

Taxel P. Osteoporosis: detection, prevention, and treatment in primary care. *Geriatrics* 1998;53:22–40.

The Writing Group for the PEPI Trial. Effects of hormone therapy on bone mineral density: results from the Postmenopausal Estrogen/Progestin Interventions (PEPI) trial. *JAMA* 1996;276(17):1389–1396.

REFERENCES

1. McClung MR, Geusens P, Miller PD, et al. Effect of risedronate on the risk of hip fracture in elderly women. *N Engl J Med* 2001;344:333–340.
2. Orwoll E, Ettinger M, Weiss S, et al. Alendronate for the treatment of osteoporosis in men. *N Engl J Med* 2000;343(9):604–610.
3. Schnitzer T, Bone HG, Crepaldi G, et al. Therapeutic equivalence of alendronate 70mg once weekly and alendronate 10mg daily in the treatment of osteoporosis. *Aging Clin Exp Res* 2000;12(1):1–12.
4. Reid IR, Brown JP, Burckhardt P, et al. Intravenous zoledronic acid in postmenopausal women with low bone mineral density. *N Engl J Med* 2002;346:653–661.
5. The MORE Investigators. Reduction of vertebral fracture risk in postmenopausal women with osteoporosis treated with raloxifene. *JAMA* 1999;282:637–645.

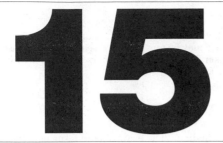

Paget's Disease of Bone (Osteitis Deformans)

Divya Shroff

INTRODUCTION

Paget's disease is the second most common bone disorder of the elderly after osteoporosis. Its incidence increases with age, and 10% of individuals >90 yrs are affected. There is a definite geographic distribution throughout the world; it commonly occurs in North America, Western Europe, and Australia but is rare in Africa, Asia, and the Middle East. Paget's disease can be monostotic (affecting one bone) or polyostotic (affecting multiple bones). Appropriate diagnosis and management can prevent serious complications such as fractures, deafness, nerve compression, and cardiac failure.

CAUSES

Pathophysiology

The etiology of Paget's disease has not been completely elucidated. Genetic and environmental factors appear to play a role. **15–30% of patients have a family history of the disease,** some with autosomal dominant inheritance. Viral infection of osteoclasts by paramyxoviruses has also been implicated.

The activity of both osteoclasts and osteoblasts is increased, as is the production of new bone matrix. This process eventually leads to dense bone that is structurally inferior and prone to fracture.

There are three phases of the disease process that play a role in clinical findings:

- An **initial osteolytic phase** of intense focal bone resorption.
- A **mixed phase** during which active bone resorption and formation are associated with the ingrowth of highly vascularized fibrous tissue. Extensive but dense tissue is formed with large amounts of blood flow, which can lead to an increase in cardiac output and shunting of blood.
- A **late sclerotic (osteoblastic) phase** during which cortical and trabecular bone encroach on the marrow space and expand the periosteal surface. The latter may cause nerve entrapment and compression.

All three phases may be active at different sites in a single patient.

History

Approximately 15% of patients are asymptomatic at presentation and are diagnosed due to an incidental finding on x-ray or elevation of alkaline phosphatase. **The most common presenting symptom is chronic pain, which may be due to bone pain or joint involvement.** The bones most commonly affected are the pelvis, spine, femur, skull, tibia, and humerus. Involvement of weight-bearing bones can present as boring or persistent bone pain, aggravated by bearing weight. Progressive and painless bowing of a long bone can also be the first symptom of the disease. Arthritis is a frequent symptom. Joints may be involved directly or may be due to subchondral involvement that results in cartilage destruction. The pain is often worse at night, in contrast to osteoarthritis. Relief with acetaminophen and NSAIDs tends to be inadequate.

Differential Diagnosis

Other causes for elevation of serum alkaline phosphatase or bone pain should be investigated. Elevated alkaline phosphatase may be due to liver disease, renal disease, hypovitaminosis D, or hyperparathyroidism. Metastatic cancer may also present with elevated alkaline phosphatase, bone pain, and osteolytic lesions.

PRESENTATION

Physical Exam

Many patients will have no physical exam findings. The exam should focus on sites of pain or known involvement and may reveal signs of bone growth or deformity. Frontal bossing and leonine facies are signs of skull involvement. Joint exam should assess for inflammation, tenderness, and limitation of motion. A thorough neurologic exam, including hearing and gait assessment, is warranted.

Diagnostic Evaluation

Bone biopsy is rarely required except to exclude sarcoma. Radiologic studies are a routine part of the evaluation.

A bone scan is more sensitive than plain films and should be obtained at the time of diagnosis to assess the extent of disease.

Plain films should be obtained at sites of pain and for baseline evaluation at asymptomatic sites found on bone scan. The most characteristic feature is the localized enlargement of bone.

Elevated lab markers correlate with disease activity and can assist with diagnosis, determining who should be treated, and assessing the response to therapy.

An elevated **alkaline phosphatase** level is a marker of increased bone formation. The serum bone-specific alkaline phosphatase concentration is a more sensitive marker of bone formation and can be a useful indicator in the management of monostotic disease.

Increased bone resorption can be measured by **urinary pyridinoline excretion** (a marker of collagen breakdown) and **urinary collagen N-telopeptide excretion** (a more sensitive test that requires morning collection as levels increase overnight). These measurements can be helpful in predominately osteolytic disease or when the alkaline phosphatase is normal.

MANAGEMENT

Complications

Fractures are the most common complication and may occur with minimal trauma. Long bones and the spine are most frequently involved.

Neurologic complications may be the presenting feature:

- The reduction in size of neural foramina can lead to compression of cranial nerves, causing nerve palsies, hearing loss, and trigeminal neuralgia.
- Brainstem and cerebellar compression and/or hydrocephalus can be due to basilar invagination.
- Compressive spinal cord and nerve root lesions can lead to radiculopathy, myelopathy, spinal stenosis, or cauda equina syndrome.
- Increased blood flow to skull bones can rarely cause shunting, leading to cerebral ischemia.

Spine disease may also cause gait abnormalities and a stooped posture. **Hearing loss** may occur as a result of ossicle involvement or nerve compression. Maxillary or mandibular involvement can result in **tooth loss or misalignment.**

Patients with Paget's disease also have an increased incidence of **inflammatory arthritides. Hyperuricemia is common and may result in gout.**

Cardiac complications include vascular calcification and high-output congestive heart failure.

Hypercalcemia can occur with immobilization (after surgery or a fracture).

Malignant sarcomatous transformation is rare and typically occurs in patients with severe polyostotic disease. A sudden rise in alkaline phosphatase, increased pain, a palpable mass, or a pathologic fracture can be a clue toward transformation. There is no effective treatment, and survival averages 6 mos. MRI findings include mixed osteoblastic and osteolytic vertebral lesions, but a bone biopsy is required for definitive diagnosis.

Treatment

The long-term goal of treatment is to return the rate of bone remodeling through antiresorptive therapy. A treatment algorithm is provided (Fig. 15-1).

Some asymptomatic patients may not require treatment but should have routine follow-up, as some will develop symptoms in the future:

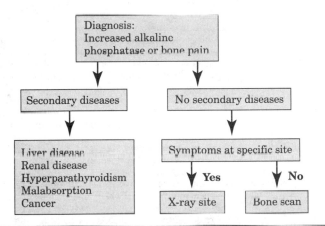

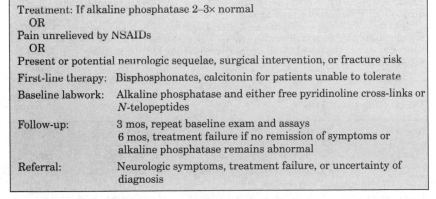

FIG. 15-1. Paget's disease treatment algorithm. (From Delmas PD, Meunier PJ. The management of Paget's disease of bone. *N Engl J Med* 1997;336:558–566, with permission.)

TABLE 15-1. BISPHOSPHONATES

Agent	Dosage	Comments
Alendronate	40 mg/day PO × 6 mos	—
Risedronate	30 mg/day PO × 3–6 mos	—
Etidronate	5–7.5 mg/kg/day PO × 6 mos	Use if patients cannot tolerate newer agents
Pamidronate	30 mg IV × 6 weekly doses or 30 mg IV × 6 monthly doses or 60 mg IV × 3 days	Use in those refractory to other medications; remission in 90% of patients for up to 3 yrs
Tiludronate	200 mg PO bid × 6 mos	

- Sites of disease with little or no risk of complications (iliac crest, sacrum, scapula)
- Minimal or no elevation of bone markers
- Short life expectancy

Bisphosphonates are the first-line treatment (Table 15-1). Their main action is to induce marked and prolonged inhibition of bone resorption by decreasing osteoclastic activity. In addition, they decrease the number of osteoclasts by decreasing their recruitment and by promoting their apoptosis. In contrast to the short-lived effects of calcitonin, disease activity remains low for many months and sometimes years after treatment with bisphosphonates is stopped. In general, the decrease in bone turnover is more pronounced and prolonged in patients with moderate disease activity (serum alkaline phosphatase levels no more than 2–4 times the upper limit of normal). The main reported side effects involve the GI tract. Ensure adequate intake of calcium (1000 mg/day) and vitamin D (800 IU/day).

Calcitonin, which decreases bone resorption, can be used for patients who cannot tolerate bisphosphonates (Table 15-2). Within a few weeks, bone pain is decreased, and within 3–6 mos, there is increased mobility, decreased blood flow to affected areas, and healed osteolytic lesions. The suppression of disease activity does not persist long after the withdrawal of calcitonin treatment (up to 1 yr). Common side effects include transient nausea and facial flushing. Up to 25% of patients develop resistance after 2–3 yrs with the development of anticalcitonin antibodies. Treatment should be discontinued after 6 mos if there is no positive response; markers rarely return to normal—usually only a therapeutic plateau is achieved.

Because of its toxicity, mithramycin (Plicamycin) is only used in severe disease that is resistant to calcitonin or bisphosphonates. Dosages can be 10–25 mg/kg for up to 10 days or 15–25 mg/kg weekly. This agent decreases bone pain and induces remission for several months.

TABLE 15-2. CALCITONIN

Agent	Dosage	Comments
Salmon calcitonin	50–100 IU SC/IM qd × 1 mo and then 3–4 days weekly × several mos	Most potent, total therapy dependent on disease activity and response
Human calcitonin	50 IU for same time period	Less likely to form antibodies
Intranasal calcitonin	200–400 IU	Use if patients cannot tolerate newer agents

Surgical Referral

Surgical consultation should be pursued for fracture repair, cord/nerve root compression treatment, and joint replacement. These patients must be treated with calcitonin or bisphosphonates for approximately 3 mos before surgery to decrease vascularity in nonemergent cases. Medications should be resumed 8 wks after surgery.

Follow-Up

The appropriate frequency and extent of follow-up for a treated patient vary according to the severity of the disease. Disease activity can be effectively monitored by measurements of serum alkaline phosphatase and urinary free pyridinoline cross-links or N-telopeptides every 6 mos. The monitoring of bone pain, articular function, and neurologic status is usually performed q3–6mos in symptomatic patients.

KEY POINTS TO REMEMBER

- Paget's disease is more common in the elderly.
- Some patients are asymptomatic and are diagnosed because of radiologic or biochemical abnormalities.
- The most common presenting symptom is chronic pain, including bone pain and arthritis.
- There are numerous possible complications, particularly fracture, neurologic compromise, and deafness.
- Baseline evaluation includes a bone scan, alkaline phosphatase, and urinary markers of bone turnover.
- Bisphosphonates are highly effective and are the first-line treatment.

REFERENCES AND SUGGESTED READINGS

Ankrom MA, Shapiro JR. Paget's disease of bone (osteitis deformans). *J Am Geriatr Soc* 1998;46:1025–1033.

Delmas PD, Meunier PJ. The management of Paget's disease of bone. *N Engl J Med* 1997;336:558–566.

Hadjipavlou AG, Gaitanis IN, Kontakis GM. Paget's disease of the bone and its management. *J Bone Joint Surg* 2002;84:160–169.

Rothschild BM. Paget's disease of the elderly. *Compr Ther* 2000;26:251–254.

16 Osteoarthritis

Rebecca M. Shepherd

INTRODUCTION

Osteoarthritis (OA) was previously thought of as part of the natural aging process, hence the term "degenerative joint disease." Now it is known to be caused by multiple factors, including genetics, biochemistry, inflammation, and mechanical forces. Because the definition, and therefore, the diagnosis, of OA can be so elusive, the NIH proposed and revised in 1994 the definition of OA:

> **Osteoarthritis** is the result of both mechanical and biologic tenets that destabilize the normal coupling of degradation and synthesis of articular cartilage and subchondral bone. It may be initiated by multiple factors including genetic, developmental, metabolic, and traumatic; OA involves all of the tissues of the diarthrodial joint. Ultimately, OA is manifested by morphologic, biochemical, molecular, and biomechanical changes of both cells and matrix, which leads to softening, fibrillation, ulceration and loss of articular cartilage, sclerosis and eburnation of subchondral bone, osteophytes, and subchondral cysts. **When clinically evident, OA is characterized by joint pain, tenderness, limitation of movement, crepitus, occasional effusion, and variable degrees of local inflammation.**

In 1995, 21 million people reported having OA, an increase from 1985 thought to be secondary to the aging population rather than due to the change in definition. **Arthritis is named the second leading cause for adults receiving Social Security disability payments.** The prevalence of OA increases with age so that, in men and women >60, the prevalence is 17% and 29.6%, respectively. The prevalence of knee OA as defined by radiographic exam of the tibiofemoral compartment was 33% in adults aged 63–93. An estimated 59.4 million Americans will be affected by some type of arthritis by the year 2020.

CAUSES

Pathophysiology

Types of OA are as follows:

- **Primary idiopathic:** either localized or generalized. The localized form affects one to two of the following joint groups (Fig. 16-1): distal interphalangeal (DIP), proximal interphalangeal (PIP), or first metacarpophalangeal (MCP) joints; cervical or lumbar spine; first metatarsophalangeal (MTP) of feet; knees; or hips. The generalized form involves three or more joint groups and is frequently associated with *Heberden's nodes,* which are bony enlargements of the DIP joints.
- **Secondary:** should be considered if patient develops OA in atypical joints such as MCP joints of the hands, wrists, ankles, shoulders, or elbows (see risk factors listed in this same section).
- **Erosive OA:** also known as **inflammatory OA;** a severe form of OA or an entity of its own. Affects the DIP and PIP joints of the hand, with negative rheumatoid factor.

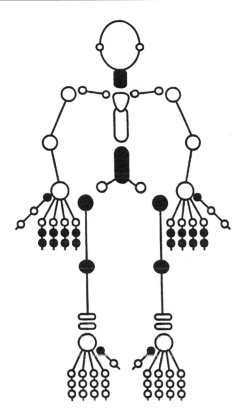

FIG. 16-1. Joint involvement in osteoarthritis.

Cartilage failure in OA is caused by an imbalance of the dynamic degradative and repair processes within the cartilage, synovium, and bone. The contributing factors are multiple and complex. The most common instigating factor is macrotrauma or repeated microtrauma to normal cartilage. As a result of injury, chondrocytes release degradative cytokines and proteases; repair efforts in response are inadequate. Also contributing are the multiple factors such as genetically defective cartilage, obesity, age, and secondary causes of OA such as endocrinopathies.

Risk factors for primary OA are as follows:

- **Age:** the prevalence of OA greatly increases with age.
- **Gender:** women experience OA more often than men.
- **Obesity:** association is present with knee and hand more than with hip.
- **High bone mass:** women with osteoporosis are less likely to have OA.
- **Mechanical factors:** repeated use of the joint leads to degeneration of the joint. This is evident in previous joint injury, repeated movement in occupational OA, such as bending and squatting, and sports-related OA.
- **Genetic:** a genetic component has been noted in subsets of OA. Knee, hip, and hand OA are particularly susceptible to genetic influence. Research suggests collagen genes and genes encoding for extracellular matrix proteins may contribute to the development of OA.

Causes of secondary OA are as follows:

- **Mechanical:** posttraumatic and postsurgical joints are apt to develop OA more frequently; congenital anomalies are also a predisposing factor, with hip dysplasia accounting for up to 25% of OA cases in white patients.
- **Inflammatory diseases:** joints affected by rheumatoid and infectious arthritis are at increased risk.
- **Metabolic disease:** acromegaly, Paget's disease [see Chap. 15, Paget's Disease of Bone (Osteitis Deformans)], Cushing's syndrome, crystal arthropathies, ochronosis, hemochromatosis, Wilson's disease, and steroid injections are predisposing factors.
- **Bleeding dyscrasias:** pathologic, such as lymphoma, or iatrogenic, such as warfarin use, can cause hemarthrosis.
- **Neuropathic joints:** seen in diabetes, syphilis, spinal cord trauma, and Charcot's joint.

Differential Diagnosis

The following diagnoses must be considered when diagnosing OA: rheumatoid arthritis; seronegative spondyloarthropathies such as psoriatic arthritis, Reiter's syndrome, ankylosing spondylitis, and enteropathic arthritis; crystalline arthropathies; infectious arthritis, including bacterial and viral etiologies; neoplastic synovitis (most common with blood dyscrasias); periarticular bursitis and tendonitis; and referred pain from a different joint.

PRESENTATION

History and Physical Exam

Patients generally present after the age of 40. The most common presenting complaint in OA is pain. The pain is mechanical in nature and worsens with activity such as walking and is alleviated with rest. As the disease progresses, stiffness can become a manifestation. **Stiffness can occur after a period of inactivity, called a gel effect,** and is alleviated within 30 mins; this is unlike rheumatoid arthritis, in which morning stiffness lasting >30 mins is a prominent symptom. OA also manifests as episodes of severe pain above the baseline chronic pain. Patients may complain of joints "locking," particularly the knees, which is due to loose material within the joint.

Exam of the suspected joint may demonstrate tenderness to palpation, usually without evidence of inflammation. Crepitus, bony enlargement, decreased range of motion, joint effusion, and osteophytes along the periphery of the joint may be found. **The joints most commonly involved are DIP and PIP joints, knees, hips, and the spine** (Fig. 16-1). **Secondary OA or another disease process should be considered if other joints are involved.**

Specific Joints

HANDS. **Hand involvement is common in OA** and occurs in women more than men. There is also a familial association. Osteoarthritic enlargements of the DIP and PIP joints are referred to as *Heberden's* and *Bouchard's nodes*, respectively. **The first MCP joint is also commonly affected in OA** and causes a squared-off appearance to the hand. Soft cysts can form on the dorsal aspect of DIP joints.

FEET. **The first MTP joint is often affected.** Bursal inflammation occurs at the medial side of the metatarsal head, called a **bunion.** Hallux rigidis occurs with limitation of dorsiflexion of the big toe, which may impede ambulation. Involvement of the subtalar joint also causes difficulty with walking.

KNEES. Tenderness along the joint line may be present, as well as crepitus on placing a hand over the patella during range of motion. Osteophytes may be palpable. The medial and lateral compartments are most often affected in OA, with cartilage loss beginning in the medial aspect of the tibiofemoral joint. Medial and lateral compartment narrowing, called **genu varus** (bow-legged) and **genu valgus** (knock-kneed), respectively, occurs secondary to malalignment. The patella may also be involved with pain and tenderness anteriorly.

HIPS. OA of the hips is most common in older patients and in men more than women. Patients describe pain in the outer groin or inner thigh area; it may also radiate to the medial knee or distal thigh, buttocks, or sciatic region. Osteoarthritic pain must be differentiated from that of trochanteric bursitis, lumbosacral or knee OA, lumbar radiculopathy, herniation, and vascular insufficiency. On exam, internal rotation is diminished, with eventual loss of extension, abduction, and flexion. Contractures occur, and shortening of the limb may be observed. A limp and eventually lordosis of the spine may develop in an effort to reduce hip pain on walking.

SPINE. Spinal involvement in OA is most common at spinal levels C5, T8, and L3, which represent the areas of greatest spinal flexibility. It can be classified as OA or spondylosis, which is OA that develops in conjunction with degenerative disc disease. OA occurs in the posterior apophyseal joints with resultant joint space narrowing, sclerosis, and osteophyte formation. Spondylosis is characterized by degenerative changes of the discs and vertebral bodies. Pain occurs from local paraspinal ligament and muscle spasm or from radicular symptoms. Radicular symptoms of the cervical spine include neck pain with radiation to the shoulders, back, and extremities and weakness and paresthesias of the upper extremities. Lumbar spine symptoms include low-back pain with radiation down to the buttocks, legs, and feet. This pain increases with exertion. **The physical exam in spinal OA is often unrevealing but may demonstrate decreased range of motion or local tenderness. Careful neurologic exam is important to detect the aforementioned radicular involvement.**

SHOULDER. **Shoulder involvement in primary OA is unusual except in elderly women,** in whom there is a rapidly progressive form. When present, OA ranges from mild discomfort to complete joint destruction. Osteophytes located along the undersurface of the acromioclavicular joint may result in rotator cuff tendonitis or tears due to the juxtaposition of tendons with the inferior portion of the acromioclavicular joint. The shoulder may rapidly deteriorate because of an aggressive form of OA that occurs in association with calcium crystalline disease (as observed in the Milwaukee shoulder syndrome).

MANAGEMENT

Diagnostic Workup

Radiographic evidence of OA is very common and does not necessarily correlate with symptomatic disease. The following features are often seen on radiographs of osteoarthritic joints: joint space narrowing, subchondral sclerosis, osteophytes at the periphery of joints, and subchondral cysts.

There are no markers for primary OA. Blood work can be obtained to rule out secondary causes of OA or differentiate between other arthritides such as rheumatoid arthritis. Rheumatoid factor, ESR, and CBC should all be normal; the **rheumatoid factor may be mildly positive in elderly patients without rheumatoid arthritis.**

Synovial fluid is noninflammatory, clear, and transparent with few white cells (<2000 WBC/mL).

The diagnosis of OA is based on the clinical picture and supported by radiologic and lab data. The American College of Rheumatology created guidelines that were originally designed as guidelines for clinical studies but can be used to assist in the diagnosis of OA. There are limitations to these guidelines in that they pertain only to certain joints, the correlation between radiographic findings and clinical presentation is highly variable, and only patients with idiopathic OA are included:

- **Knee:** knee pain and osteophytes and one of the following: age >50, crepitus on motion, or stiffness lasting <30 mins.
- **Hand:** hand pain, aching, or stiffness and at least three of the following: hard tissue enlargement of >1 of the selected joints (second and third DIP or PIP and the first carpometacarpal joint of each hand), hard tissue enlargement of >1 DIP joints, deformity of at least 1 of 10 selected joints, or <3 swollen MCP joints.
- **Hip:** hip pain and at least two of the following: ESR <20 mm/hr, radiographic acetabular or femoral osteophytes, or radiographic joint space narrowing.

Treatment and Follow-Up

The treatment of OA should be a multimodal approach to reduce pain and disability and improve quality of life. Treatment is not necessary during the asymptomatic phase of OA.

Nonpharmacologic Approach

• Reduction of stress and load on the joint.
• Strengthening of surrounding periarticular muscles and maintaining joint stability and flexibility; this can be accomplished with the aid of a trained physical therapist. Occupational therapy may be useful in symptomatic OA of the hand.
• Weight reduction.
• Patient education and self-help groups: Arthritis Foundation 1-800-283-7800; http://www.arthritis.org.

Pharmacologic Therapies

ANALGESICS. **Topical analgesics,** such as capsaicin and salicylate, are effective in reducing pain in specific joints such as knee, shoulder, elbow, and hand. They are most effective when used for intermittent isolated flares in those who cannot tolerate PO agents.

ACETAMINOPHEN. Acetaminophen is indicated for pain control in those whom nonpharmacologic agents have not worked. Dosing is safe at <4000 g PO per day (or <2 g in patients with liver failure or alcohol use). This analgesic has no antiinflammatory effects. Many studies have confirmed the benefit of acetaminophen in treating OA, but whether it is equivalent to NSAIDs is controversial. Some studies demonstrate equivalent results in patient satisfaction, whereas others show a patient preference for NSAIDs. Hepatotoxicity is the most common side effect and occurs in those with concurrent liver damage from other processes such as alcohol and chronic hepatitis C.

NSAIDS. The role of nonselective NSAIDs has been long-standing and invaluable in the treatment of OA. Recent studies have demonstrated that selective cyclooxygenase (COX)-2 inhibitors are equally effective with fewer GI side effects. The role of gastroprotective agents with NSAIDs is also discussed later. At low doses (e.g., ibuprofen, 1200 mg PO qd), NSAIDs act as an analgesic by inhibiting prostaglandin sensitization of peripheral pain receptors. At higher doses (e.g., ibuprofen, 2400 mg PO per day), NSAIDs inhibit production of COX, which catalyzes the production of prostaglandins from arachidonic acid. Many different NSAIDs can be used to control pain in patients with OA. Choosing an appropriate NSAID depends on such factors as efficacy, cost, frequency of dosing, prior adverse reactions, and comorbidities such as peptic ulcer disease or renal dysfunction. No specific class of NSAID is known to be superior to the others.

The following considerations may be helpful in prescribing an effective NSAID:

• A short-acting NSAID taken prn is appropriate for episodic pain. Continuous therapy is indicated if prn dosing does not control the pain.
• If pain control is not adequate, the dose of a specific NSAID should be maximized before declaring treatment failure; 2–4 wks is a sufficient trial period.
• **The elderly are particularly susceptible to the toxicity of NSAIDs** such as GI upset and bleeding; renal impairment and sodium retention in those with renal disease, heart failure, or diuretic use; and neurologic dysfunction.

PROTECTION AGAINST GI TOXICITY. (See *Washington Manual Gastroenterology Subspecialty Consult.*) Several trials recently have investigated the use of gastroprotective agents in patients who take NSAIDs. In the OMNIUM study [1], treatment of ulcers, erosions, and gastric symptoms were similar between the group using misoprostol (Cytotec) and those using 20 mg and 40 mg omeprazole (Prilosec). Secondary prevention or "maintenance" was more successful with the omeprazole arm. The ASTRONAUT study demonstrated that omeprazole healed and prevented relapse in patients with both gastric and duodenal ulcers [2]. Two previous trials have demonstrated that there is a reduction in duodenal, but not gastric, ulcers with the use of ranitidine (Zantac). The trials can be used to guide primary preventive therapy in high-risk patients, although large controlled trials to date focus on secondary prevention.

SELECTIVE COX-2 INHIBITORS. **Selective COX-2 inhibitors** spare COX-1, which accounts for decreased GI toxicity. Celecoxib (Celebrex), rofecoxib (Vioxx), and valdecoxib (Bextra) have been approved for the treatment of OA. Studies such as the VIGOR [3] and CLASS [4] trials demonstrate fewer GI complications of selective COX-2 inhibitors compared to nonselective inhibitors. **They should not be used in cases of renal disease, heart failure, or volume depletion.**

OPIATES. Although not routinely used, opiates can give significant relief to patients in whom NSAIDs are contraindicated and surgery is not an option.

CORTICOSTEROIDS. There is no indication for oral use of corticosteroids in OA. **Steroid injections are indicated in patients who have pain in one or two joints and inadequate response to NSAIDs or inability to take NSAIDs.** Steroids reduce biochemical turnover of the cartilage and osteophyte formation in animal models. Injections should be given only when infection is not suspected. Corticosteroids are frequently mixed with lidocaine and injected in crystalline form. The amount of steroid injected depends on the size of the joint. Intraarticular injections of the hips generally should not be undertaken unless under fluoroscopic guidance. Injections should only be given 3 or 4 times yearly per joint.

Intraarticular injection of **hyaluronate** into the knee joint can be effective in decreasing pain for several months. Two forms are currently available, Hyalgan (sodium hyaluronate) and Synvisc (hylan G-F 20), which can be injected intraarticularly in weekly doses for 3 and 5 wks, respectively. Intraarticular hyaluronate is FDA approved for knees.

Arthroscopic irrigation may be indicated in patients who have OA of the knee or shoulder that is not controlled with NSAIDs or intraarticular corticosteroids. The procedure involves irrigating the joint with sterile normal saline through a closed needle to remove debris and crystalline material. The procedure is best performed with visual guidance to irrigate all compartments of the knee.

Referral to the surgical specialists should be undertaken when conservative measures are no longer effective at relieving pain or the joint becomes unstable. The aim of surgical intervention is to relieve pain and improve function of the joint via fusion or replacement of joint with prostheses. Arthroplasty, or total joint replacement, provides significant pain relief; it is only undertaken in those patients who are medically stable enough to undergo surgical intervention and strenuous rehabilitation. Prostheses are expected to last 15 yrs, although obesity and higher activity levels increase the chance of prosthetic failure.

KEY POINTS TO REMEMBER

- OA is very prevalent in the elderly and manifests with symptoms of mechanical joint pain.
- Osteoarthritis can contribute to falls, functional decline, and driving impairment in the older adult.
- The joints most commonly involved are DIP and PIP joints, knees, hips, and spine.
- OA affects PIP, DIP, and first MCP joints of hands.
- Surgical referral is indicated with uncontrollable pain or joint instability.
- The elderly are most susceptible to the toxicity of NSAIDs, including gastroduodenal ulcers, renal dysfunction, hypertension, and edema.
- Nonpharmacologic approaches are useful and should be reinforced at each patient encounter.

SUGGESTED READING

Altman R, Alarcon G, Appelrouth D, et al. The American College of Rheumatology criteria for the classification and reporting of osteoarthritis of the hip. *Arthritis Rheum* 1991;34:505.

Altman R, Alarcon G, Appelrouth D, et al. The American College of Rheumatology criteria for the classification and reporting of osteoarthritis of the hand. *Arthritis Rheum* 1990;33:1601.

Bombardier C, Laine L, Reicin A, et al. Comparison of upper gastrointestinal toxicity of rofecoxib and naproxen in patients with rheumatoid arthritis. *N Engl J Med* 2000;343:1520.

Creamer P, Hochberg MC. Osteoarthritis. *Lancet* 1997;350:503.

Hawkey CJ, Karrasch JA, Szczepanski L, et al. Omeprazole compared with misoprostol for ulcers associated with nonsteroidal antiinflammatory drugs. *N Engl J Med* 1998;338:727.

MacLean CH. Quality indicators for the management of osteoarthritis in vulnerable elders. *Ann Intern Med* 2001;135:711–721.

Moskowitz RW. Clinical and laboratory findings in osteoarthritis. In: Koopman WJ, ed. *Arthritis and allied conditions*. Baltimore: Williams & Wilkins, 1997:1985–2011.

The management of persistent pain in older persons: AGS panel on persistent pain in older persons. *J Am Geriatr Soc* 2002;50:205–224.

National Arthritis Data Workgroup. Arthritis prevalence and activity limitation— United States, 1990. *MMWR Morb Mortal Wkly Rep* 1994;43:433.

Recommendations for the medical management of osteoarthritis of the hip and knee: 2000 update. American College of Rheumatology Subcommittee on Osteoarthritis Guidelines. *Arthritis Rheum* 2000;43:1905–1915.

Solomon L. Clinical features of osteoarthritis. In: Kelley WN, Hams ED, Ruddy S, et al., eds. *Textbook of rheumatology*. Philadelphia: WB Saunders, 1996:1383.

Yeomans ND, Tulassay Z, Juhasz L, et al. A comparison of omeprazole with ranitidine for ulcers associated with nonsteroidal antiinflammatory drugs. *N Engl J Med* 1998;338:719.

REFERENCES

1. Hawkey CJ, Karrasch JA, Szczepanski L, et al. Omeprazole compared with misoprostol for ulcers associated with nonsteroidal antiinflammatory drugs. *N Engl J Med* 1998;338:727.
2. Yeomans ND, Tulassay Z, Juhasz L, et al. A comparison of omeprazole with ranitidine for ulcers Associated with nonsteroidal antiinflammatory drugs. *N Engl J Med* 1998;338:719.
3. Bombardier C, Laine L, Reicin A, et al. Comparison of upper gastrointestinal toxicity of rofecoxib and naproxen in patients with rheumatoid arthritis. *N Engl J Med* 2000;343:1520.
4. Silverstein FE, Faich G, Goldstein JL, et al. Gastrointestinal toxicity with celecoxib vs nonsteroidal anti-inflammatory drugs for osteoarthritis and rheumatoid arthritis: the CLASS study: a randomized controlled trial. Celecoxib Long-Term Arthritis Safety Study. *JAMA* 2000;284:1247–1255.

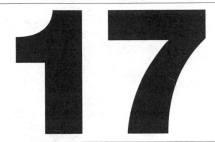

Giant Cell Arteritis and Polymyalgia Rheumatica

Ulker Tok

INTRODUCTION

Giant cell arteritis (GCA), or **temporal arteritis,** is defined by the Chapel Hill Consensus conference as a granulomatous arteritis of the aorta and its major branches, with a predilection for the extracranial branches of the carotid artery [1]. **It often involves the temporal artery and usually occurs in individuals >50 yrs. Polymyalgia rheumatica (PMR) is a syndrome classically characterized by symmetric aching and morning stiffness in the shoulder and hip girdles, neck, and torso in patients >50 yrs.** A close relationship exists between PMR and GCA. Although the precise nature of the association is not fully understood, they are considered by some investigators to be different phases of the same disease. PMR occurs in 50% of patients with GCA, whereas approximately 15% of patients with PMR develop GCA.

GCA is relatively common in Europe and the United States with an annual incidence of 0.49–27.3/100,000 persons aged ≥ 50 yrs. Autopsy studies have suggested a more common occurrence of GCA. The incidence of PMR was 52.5/100,000 persons >50 yrs in one study. **Women are affected twice as often as men.** Both GCA and PMR are more common in those with northern European ancestry.

CAUSES

Pathophysiology

Increased incidence of the two disorders after age 50 yrs implies a relationship to aging. Reports on familial aggregation and an apparent increased incidence in persons from northern Europe and the United States suggest a genetic predisposition. Patients with PMR and GCA share a sequence polymorphism in the HLA-DRB1 gene, which may be linked to antigen selection and presentation. Both humoral and cellular immune systems have been implicated in pathogenesis. Whether one develops PMR or GCA may depend on the cytokines that are activated. There is evidence that patients with PMR also have vascular involvement.

The vasculitis in GCA tends to be patchy. **The most severely affected arteries are the superficial temporal, vertebral, ophthalmic, and posterior ciliary arteries.** Intimal thickening with prominent cellular infiltration is usually present. Necrosis of arterial walls and granulomas may also be seen. Predominant cells are lymphocytes and multinucleated giant cells; neutrophils are rare.

Pathologic exam of joints with PMR may show lymphocytic synovitis. Synovial fluid analysis may be consistent with mild inflammation.

Differential Diagnosis

A few patients with findings of PMR develop persistent joint pain and swelling, which mimics seronegative rheumatoid arthritis. PMR may also mimic hypothyroidism, fibromyalgia, polymyositis, or other chronic inflammatory states such as bacterial endocarditis.

The differential diagnosis of GCA includes Takayasu arteritis. Takayasu arteritis begins at a young age, does not commonly involve branches of the external carotid artery, and has not been demonstrated to involve the temporal artery. In rare cases, polyarteritis nodosa or Wegener's granulomatosis may involve the temporal artery. Occasionally, amyloidosis affects the temporal arteries and causes jaw and arm claudication.

PRESENTATION

History and Physical Exam

Onset for both GCA and PMR may be abrupt or insidious; symptoms are usually present for weeks or months before the diagnosis is established. PMR is classically characterized by **symmetric aching and morning stiffness in the shoulder and hip girdles, neck, and torso.** Fatigue, malaise, anorexia, weight loss, and low-grade fever may also occur. Synovitis in peripheral joints that promptly resolves with steroid treatment may be seen, making PMR difficult to distinguish from rheumatoid arthritis. Swelling and pitting edema over the hands, wrists, ankles, and top of the feet and carpal tunnel syndrome may also be present. Joint exam shows decreased active range of motion of the shoulders, neck, and hips owing to pain. **Muscle strength is usually normal.**

Headache is the most common initial symptom of GCA. The severity and location are variable. **Scalp tenderness** is also common and may be localized to temporal or occipital arteries or may be diffuse. The temporal arteries may be thickened, erythematous, and tender. **Vision loss occurs in approximately 15% of patients and may be an early symptom.** It results from ischemic optic neuropathy secondary to the involvement of ophthalmic and posterior ciliary arteries. It is abrupt and painless. Once established, the visual deficit is usually permanent. Funduscopy shows a pale disc with blurred margins consistent with ischemic optic neuropathy. **Involvement of the facial artery may result in pain and spasm with mastication known as jaw claudication.**

Involvement of the aortic arch and its branches occurs in 10–15% of patients and may cause reduced BP in one or both arms, arm claudication, and focal cerebral ischemia. Peripheral neuropathy or involvement of the skin, intracranial vessels, kidneys, or lungs rarely occurs.

MANAGEMENT

Diagnostic Workup

The American College of Rheumatology criteria for the classification of GCA requires three of the following five [2]:

1. Age of onset >50 yrs
2. New headache
3. Temporal artery tenderness or decreased pulsation unrelated to atherosclerotic disease
4. ESR >50 mm/hr
5. Arterial biopsy specimen showing vasculitis with mononuclear cell infiltration, granulomatous inflammation, or multinucleated giant cells

GCA should be suspected in patients >50 yrs who develop a new type of headache, jaw claudication, transient or sudden loss of vision, unexplained prolonged fever or anemia, high sedimentation rate, and PMR.

Temporal artery biopsies should be performed in patients with suspected GCA or those with PMR who have symptoms or signs suggestive of GCA. To increase the chances that a biopsy will demonstrate vasculitis, the biopsy should be several centimeters long and include a section of a palpable abnormality if present. **If the biopsy of one temporal artery is negative, contralateral biopsy should be done if the clinical suspicion is high.** Clinical and lab data are rarely helpful in predicting the results of a biopsy. A properly performed temporal artery biopsy defines the need for corticosteroid therapy in 90% of cases.

The American College of Rheumatology does not have a set of classification criteria for PMR. The diagnosis of PMR is clinical and should be considered in elderly patients with symmetric aching and morning stiffness in the shoulder and hip girdles, neck, and torso. The ESR is classically elevated and can exceed 100 mm/hr, but values <40 mm/hr may be seen in a few patients. Elevated C-reactive protein (CRP) levels may be more sensitive than the ESR. Normocytic normochromic anemia of chronic inflammation and thrombocytosis may be seen; leukocyte and differential counts are generally normal. Rheumatoid factor and antinuclear antibodies are usually negative. Elevated hepatic enzymes occur in 20–30% of patients. Serum creatine kinase is normal. **Tissue diagnosis of PMR is not necessary.**

Treatment and Follow-Up

PMR is characterized by a prompt response to low-dose steroids. Depending on a patient's weight and symptoms, **oral prednisone,** 7.5–20 mg qd, can be tried. The dose is increased to a maximum of 20 mg qd if symptoms are not well controlled within 1 wk. The effective dose should be maintained for 4 wks after the aching and stiffness have resolved. The dose is then reduced by 10% q2–4wks until the minimum dose that suppresses symptoms is reached. Once the dose is 10 mg qd or lower, it is reduced not faster than 1 mg/mo. **NSAIDs** may be used for mild disease. Initial ESR and CRP and initial responses to therapy provide useful prognostic information. Those patients with initial and persistently elevated high ESR and CRP levels after 1 mo of therapy are likely to require treatment for extended periods of time. Steroids may be tapered successfully in some patients within 1 yr. Most require treatment for 3–4 yrs, but withdrawal of steroids after 2 yrs is worth attempting. **In most patients, PMR improves, and steroid therapy can eventually be discontinued.** There is no evidence that patients with PMR have increased mortality compared to the general population.

  Patients strongly suspected of having GCA, especially those with impending vascular complications such as vision loss, should be started on corticosteroids. Oral prednisone, 40–60 mg qd, in single or divided doses is adequate. Inflammatory changes on biopsy specimens may be present for weeks after steroids are started. **Pulse IV methylprednisolone** (Solu-Medrol), 1000 mg qd, for 3 days followed by **daily PO prednisone,** 40–60 mg qd, should be used in patients with vision loss. 1 mo after symptoms resolve, steroid tapering as outlined earlier for PMR should begin. **ESR may not return to normal and should not be used as the only measure of disease activity.** It may be necessary to continue prednisone, 10–20 mg qd, for several months before further reductions are tried. GCA tends to last several months to years, and steroids can eventually be reduced or discontinued. Some patients may require longer duration of therapy.

  Steroid-sparing drugs such as **methotrexate** (Rheumatrex) or **azathioprine** (Imuran) may be used in those patients at increased risk for steroid-related side effects, but strong evidence of efficacy is lacking.

  Follow-up of GCA requires assessment of extracranial large-vessel involvement and its sequelae, such as aortic dissection; renal artery stenosis; HTN; coronary artery disease; and subclavian, iliac, or femoral artery stenosis. Patients with PMR should be evaluated and observed for evidence of GCA.

KEY POINTS TO REMEMBER

- GCA is unusual in patients <50 yrs.
- PMR may be difficult to distinguish from rheumatoid arthritis.
- GCA may be a cause of fever of unknown origin or failure to thrive in the elderly.
- If a diagnosis of GCA is strongly suspected, steroid therapy should be started empirically while arrangements are made for biopsy.

SUGGESTED READING

Barilla-LaBarca ML, Lenschow DJ, Brasington RD. Polymyalgia rheumatica/temporal arteritis: recent advances. *Curr Rheum Report* 2002;4:39–46.

Gonzales-Gay MA, Garcia-Porrua C, Salvarini C, et al. Diagnostic approach in a patient with polymyalgia. *Clin Exp Rheumatol* 1999;17:276–278.

Hunder GC. Giant cell arteritis and polymyalgia rheumatica. *Med Clin North Am* 1997;81:195–219.

Jennette JC, Falk RJ, Andrassy K. Nomenclature of systemic vasculitides: proposal of an international consensus conference. *Arthritis Rheum* 1994;37:187–192.

Salvarini C, Macchioni P, Bioardi L. Polymyalgia rheumatica. *Lancet* 1997;350:43–47.

Smetana GW, Shmerling RH. Does this patient have temporal arteritis? *JAMA* 2002;287:92–101.

Weyand CM. The pathogenesis of giant cell arteritis. *J Rheumatol* 2000;27:517–522.

REFERENCES

1. Jennette JC, Falk RJ, Andrassy K, et al. Nomenclature of systemic vasculitides: the proposal of an international consesus conference. *Arthritis Rheum* 1994; 37:187–192.

2. Hunder GC, Bloch DA, Michel BA, et al. The American College of Rheumatology 1990 criteria for the classification of giant cell arteritis. *Arthritis Rheum* 1990; 33:1122–1128.

Thyroid Disease in the Geriatric Patient

Divya Shroff and
Kyle C. Moylan

INTRODUCTION

The diagnosis of thyroid dysfunction in the geriatric population can be challenging. Many of the symptoms associated with thyroid disease are nonspecific and are frequently encountered in the elderly population. These symptoms could be attributed to aging itself, other disease processes, or medications. The numerous medications these patients are prescribed can also make the interpretation of thyroid tests difficult (Table 18-1). Likewise, the presence of an acute illness may also influence the results of thyroid tests. In clinical practice, physicians must decide which elderly patients should be screened for thyroid dysfunction.

THE AGING THYROID GLAND

The thyroid gland increases in nodularity with age. The weight, uptake of iodine, and follicular volume all decrease, with a resulting decrease in production of T_4. Due to a reduction in peripheral clearance, serum levels of T_4 remain unchanged. Serum T_3 values may be lower in the elderly due to decreasing peripheral deiodination and conversion of T_4 to T_3.

SCREENING GERIATRIC OUTPATIENTS FOR THYROID DYSFUNCTION

It makes sense to screen for thyroid dysfunction in the geriatric population for several reasons. **Thyroid dysfunction is common, affecting 20% of outpatients >65 yrs, and** has serious consequences. It is treatable, and a quick, noninvasive screening test is available (the TSH assay). Nevertheless, there is controversy surrounding which patients should be routinely screened; there have been several practice guidelines published by different organizations, and each recommends different criteria [1]. All of the guidelines recognize that thyroid disease is much more common in women, and thus the yield of screening women is higher. **A reasonable approach is to screen all women >55 yrs with a TSH level and all adults >75 yrs with a TSH and T_4 level.** In the frail elderly, a normal TSH may not exclude thyroid dysfunction. An abnormal TSH warrants follow-up testing of the serum total or free T_4 level.

It should be noted that the preceding discussion is focused on screening a population of healthy outpatients. There are frequently specific clinical signs and symptoms that raise the question of thyroid disease and deserve lab investigation. Table 18-2 **lists conditions in the elderly that may warrant thyroid testing.**

SCREENING HOSPITALIZED PATIENTS FOR THYROID DISEASE

As with any test, physicians must be aware of the limitations of a diagnostic test. The TSH is a very sensitive screening test for thyroid dysfunction, but it can be misinterpreted in patients with acute illnesses or with use of certain medications. **Nonthyroidal illnesses result in thyroid function test abnormalities proportional to the severity of the illness.** There are also thyroid test abnormalities that result during the recovery phase of an acute illness. The resulting situation is as follows: The more acutely ill the patient, the more likely it is that thyroid function tests will be abnormal

TABLE 18-1. MEDICATIONS THAT AFFECT THYROID FUNCTION

Drugs that decrease TSH secretion
  Dopamine
  Glucocorticoids
  Octreotide
Drugs that decrease thyroid hormone secretion
  Lithium
  Iodide
  Amiodarone
  Aminoglutethimide
Drugs that increase thyroid hormone secretion
  Iodide
  Amiodarone
Drugs that decrease T_4 absorption
  Colestipol
  Cholestyramine
  Aluminum hydroxide
  Ferrous sulfate
  Sucralfate
Drugs that increase serum thyroid–binding globulin concentration
  Estrogens
  Tamoxifen
  Heroin
  Methadone
  Mitotane
  Fluorouracil
Drugs that decrease serum thyroid–binding globulin concentration
  Androgens
  Anabolic steroids (e.g., danazol)
  Slow-release nicotinic acid
  Glucocorticoids
Drugs that displace thyroid hormone from protein-binding sites
  Furosemide
  Fenclofenac
  Mefenamic acid
  Salicylates
Drugs that alter thyroid hormone metabolism
  Phenobarbital
  Rifampin
  Phenytoin
  Carbamazepine
  Propylthiouracil
  Amiodarone
  Beta-adrenergic antagonist drugs
  Glucocorticoids

TABLE 18-2. MEDICAL CONDITIONS ASSOCIATED WITH THYROID DISEASE

Atrial fibrillation	Depression
Congestive heart failure	Hyperlipidemia
Myopathy	Osteoporosis
Carpal tunnel syndrome	Anemia
Cognitive dysfunction	Hyponatremia

and difficult to interpret. Consideration should be given to **delay screening for thyroid dysfunction until after the patient has recovered,** unless it seems that the acute illness is a direct result of a thyroidal illness (i.e., thyroid storm or myxedema) or contributing to the illness. Because of its long half-life (10–15 days), the T_4 is useful in the diagnosis of thyroid dysfunction in acute illness.

APPROACH TO HYPOTHYROIDISM IN THE GERIATRIC PATIENT

There is a high prevalence of hypothyroidism in patients >60 yrs, primarily affecting women. The **most common cause** in this age group is **autoimmune thyroid disease.** Other etiologies include previous thyroid surgery or radioiodine therapy, a history of Graves' disease, and iodine-containing drugs (i.e., amiodarone). Most cases of myxedema coma occur in patients >60 yrs.

Clinical Findings

Classic hypothyroid symptoms are often absent in this age group, whereas some manifestations could mistakenly be attributed to aging or another illness. Table 18-3 compares the clinical features of overt hypothyroidism in elderly vs. young patients.

TABLE 18-3. COMPARISON OF CLINICAL FEATURES OF HYPOTHYROIDISM IN ELDERLY VS. YOUNG PATIENTS

Symptoms and signs	Elderly (≥70 yrs) (%)	Young (≤55 yrs) (%)
Fatigue	68	83
Weakness	53	67
Cold intolerance	35	65
Dry skin	35	45
Constipation	33	41
Reduced hearing	32	25
Depression	28	52
Weight gain	24	59
Hypoactive reflexes	24	31
Muscle cramps	20	55
Paresthesia	18	61
Bradycardia	12	19
Hair loss	12	28
Disorientation	9	0

Modified from Hassani S, Hershman J. Thyroid diseases. In: Hazzard WR, ed. *Principles of geriatric medicine and gerontology*, 4th ed. New York: McGraw-Hill, 1999.

Neurologic, psychiatric, and vague symptoms predominate. Other associated conditions that could be related include open angle glaucoma, anemia, hypercholesterolemia, hyponatremia, and myopathy (including an elevated creatine phosphokinase).

Physical Exam

The physical exam may be unhelpful. A goiter is often nonpalpable. However, patients may exhibit bradycardia, delayed relaxation of deep tendon reflexes, myxedema, weakness, and cool, dry skin.

Diagnosis

Diagnosis is essentially the same as with the younger population: an elevated TSH (>5 mU/mL) with low total or free T_4 confirms the diagnosis.

Treatment

Treatment is also the same as with younger patients:

L-thyroxine should be started at 50–100 µg PO per day and increased q4–6wks by 25 µg PO per day. With this treatment, patients are usually euthyroid in 6–8 wks. Lifelong therapy with twice yearly TSH measurement is the standard recommendation.

Drugs such as ferrous sulfate, cholestyramine, sucralfate, and aluminum hydroxide antacids interfere with T_4 absorption in the GI tract; therefore, these medications should be given 4 hrs apart. Phenytoin (Dilantin), carbamazepine, estrogens, and rifampin increase the dose requirement of T_4.

Elderly patients are very sensitive to iatrogenic hyperthyroidism, which can be exhibited by palpitations, a fine tremor, difficulty concentrating, or other symptoms of hyperthyroidism (see Clinical Findings). This is diagnosed by a suppressed TSH level. In this setting, the medication should be held for 1 wk and restarted at a lower dose.

Patients with **ischemic heart disease** should be closely monitored, because T_4 replacement can precipitate angina symptoms or a myocardial infarction. However, in most patients, T_4 replacement improves cardiac output and coronary perfusion.

Patients with **myxedema** coma should be treated with steroids until coexistent adrenal insufficiency is excluded.

SUBCLINICAL HYPOTHYROIDISM

Subclinical hypothyroidism refers to patients with an elevated TSH (usually mildly elevated) combined with a normal free T_4 level. **It is a common geriatric condition** and is seen in 15% of women >65 yrs. There is no consensus regarding which patients should be treated (see Suggested Reading: Cooper, 2001).

Management should consist of confirming the findings of an elevated TSH and a normal free T_4 while considering the patient's clinical situation and medications (these findings are consistent with recovery from an acute illness). **Send a test for antibodies against thyroperoxidase and a lipid panel.** Patients with positive antibodies are usually treated because of a high conversion rate to overt hypothyroidism; patients with an elevated low-density lipoprotein or total cholesterol are frequently treated in an effort to improve lipid profiles. Untreated patients should be monitored on a yearly basis.

APPROACH TO HYPERTHYROIDISM IN THE GERIATRIC PATIENT

15–25% of total cases of hyperthyroidism are people >65 yrs. Men and women are equally affected. Common etiologies include toxic multinodular goiter, solitary toxic adenoma, amiodarone, and Graves' disease.

Clinical Findings

Geriatric patients have fewer classic symptoms of hyperthyroidism. See Table 18-4 for a comparison of the clinical features of elderly and young patients. **The most**

TABLE 18-4. COMPARISON OF CLINICAL FEATURES OF HYPERTHYROIDISM IN ELDERLY VS. YOUNG PATIENTS

Symptoms and signs	Elderly (>70 yrs) (%)	Young (<50 yrs) (%)
Tachycardia	71	96
Fatigue	56	84
Weight loss	50	51
Tremor	44	84
Dyspnea	41	56
Apathy	41	25
Anorexia	32	4
Nervousness	31	84
Hyperactive reflexes	28	96
Weakness	27	61
Depression	24	22
Increased sweating	24	95
Diarrhea	18	43
Confusion	16	0
Heat intolerance	15	92
Constipation	15	0

Modified from Hassani S, Hershman J. Thyroid diseases. In: Hazzard WR, ed. *Principles of geriatric medicine and gerontology*, 4th ed. New York: McGraw-Hill, 1999.

common symptoms are tachycardia (including atrial fibrillation), fatigue, weight loss, and tremor. The term **apathetic hyperthyroidism** describes the elderly patient with few or no symptoms of hyperthyroidism, frequently presenting with lethargy and fatigue.

Physical Findings

Physical findings are also **frequently absent.** Goiter is only present in one-half of the elderly patients compared to >90% of young patients. Hyperactive reflexes are usually not present. Proximal muscle weakness may be present (can the patient rise from a chair without using his or her arms?).

Diagnosis and Treatment

Diagnosis and treatment are **the same as for younger patients.** Antithyroid drugs should be given to relatively healthy geriatric patients, especially those with large goiters or thyrotoxicosis, to achieve a euthyroid state before radioactive iodine therapy (the treatment of choice). Beta-adrenergic symptoms can be managed with propranolol.

SUBCLINICAL HYPERTHYROIDISM

Subclinical hyperthyroidism is characterized by a suppressed TSH (<0.1 µU/mL) with normal free T_4 levels. It is much less common in the geriatric population than subclinical hypothyroidism (after excluding iatrogenic cases). **Usually, the patients are asymptomatic, although they are more prone to osteoporosis and atrial fibrillation.**

Differential Diagnosis

Differential diagnosis includes nonthyroidal illness, medications (dopamine and exogenous glucocorticoids), recovery from hyperthyroidism treatment, hypothalamic pituitary disease, and T_3 toxicosis.

Management

Check bone densitometry in postmenopausal women. Consider radioiodine therapy for patients with osteoporosis, atrial fibrillation (may not be curative), or possible symptomatic hyperthyroidism. Estrogen and calcium may attenuate bone mineral loss in postmenopausal women (see Chap. 13, Sex Hormone Therapy in the Elderly Woman).

KEY POINTS TO REMEMBER

* Thyroid disease affects 20% of outpatients >65 yrs. Most cases of myxedema coma occur in the elderly.
* Screening for thyroid disease is appropriate for many asymptomatic elderly patients as well as in those with certain medical conditions associated with thyroid dysfunction.
* Symptoms and lab studies of thyroid disease in the elderly are different than their younger counterparts. Classic symptoms are less prominent.
* Medications frequently used in the elderly may alter thyroid function and testing.
* Some patients with subclinical thyroid dysfunction may require treatment.

SUGGESTED READING

Attia J, et al. Diagnosis of thyroid disease in hospitalized patients: a systematic review. *Arch Intern Med* 1999;159:658–665.

Cooper DS. Subclinical hypothyroidism. *N Engl J Med* 2001;345:260–265.

Hassani S, Hershman J. Thyroid diseases. In: Hazzard WR, ed. *Principles of geriatric medicine and gerontology*, 4th ed. New York: McGraw-Hill, 1999.

Rae P, Farrar J, Beckett G, et al. Fortnightly review: assessment of thyroid status in elderly people. *BMJ* 1993;307:177–180.

Surks MI, Sievert, R. Drug therapy: drugs and thyroid function. *N Engl J Med* 1995;333:1688–1694.

Toft AD. Subclinical hyperthyroidism. *N Engl J Med* 2001;345:512–516.

REFERENCE

1. Arbelle J, Porath A. Practice guidelines for the detection and management of thyroid dysfunction. A comparative review of the recommendations. *Clin Endocrinol* 1999;51:11–18.

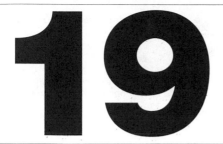

Ophthalmology and Geriatrics

Susan M. Culican

OCULAR HEALTH MAINTENANCE

A routine eye exam should be a part of any geriatric health maintenance plan. A biannual screening exam is usually sufficient for patients with no visual complaints (annual exam for diabetics). In these cases, the goal is to detect pathology before it threatens vision. Patients with visual complaints of any kind should be followed regularly by an ophthalmologist. Visual impairment can contribute to sensory deprivation, delirium, functional decline, motor vehicle collisions, and falls. More than one-half of the legally blind patients in the United States are >65 yrs.

AGE-RELATED CHANGES

During normal aging, there are a number of changes that occur in the eye that patients may or may not notice.

Anterior Segment

Patients may notice the development of arcus senilus, which is easily seen as a white or bluish ring of opacification on the cornea. There is no clinical significance or correlation with serum lipid levels.

There is also an age-related decrease in the amount and quality of the tear film that is produced by the lacrimal glands. Older patients frequently complain of "dry eye" or irritated eyes. Typically, this is more of a nuisance than a visually threatening problem, but in severe cases (or in Sjögren's syndrome) the corneal health may be compromised. **Artificial tears often relieve symptoms.** An ophthalmologist should evaluate refractory cases.

Lenticular Changes

All patients develop lenticular changes, including presbyopia and cataract.

Most people develop presbyopia around the age of 44 yrs. Presbyopia is the lack of ability of the native lens to accommodate. This requires reading glasses in emmetropic patients or bifocals in people requiring a distance correction. The amount of accommodation that is lost is linear over a period of approximately 12 yrs.

Cataracts are associated with increasing age. All patients develop some mild cataractous change in their lenses as they age, as the lens can no longer eliminate the waste products and cellular debris. Whether the cataract becomes visually significant, however, depends on family history, comorbidities such as diabetes, use of cataract-inducing medications, or prior trauma (surgical or accidental). This condition has significant morbidity and mortality associated with it and requires evaluation. **Older individuals with cataracts have an elevated risk of motor vehicle collision** when compared to age- and activity-matched controls (ICOM study) [1]. The risk can be substantially reduced by successful surgical treatment. Surgery is indicated for vision loss that is impacting daily function when removal of the cataract is likely to result in visual improvement. **>85% of patients undergoing cata-**

ract surgery report improved vision, and cataract surgery is the most frequently performed operation in the geriatric population.

Posterior Segment

The vitreous in young people is a dense gelatinous substance, becoming progressively more liquefied with age (syneresis). The most common symptom that patients report related to vitreous syneresis is the presence of **"floaters,"** but of concern is the fact that this syneresis can predispose patients to retinal tears, breaks, and detachments.

Visual Changes

Aging is associated with decreased contrast sensitivity and restriction of the functional field of vision. Patients may require increased light intensity for adequate vision.

EYE EXAM

All eye exams start with the 5 "vital signs" of ophthalmology:

- **Visual acuity** (to assess optical axis as well as macular function) (see Appendix J for Rosenbaum chart)
- **Pupil exam** (to detect evidence of optic neuropathy)
- **Tonometry** (or pressure in the eye)
- **Motility**
- **Visual field**

The physical exam includes three components:

- The external exam describes problems that can be identified by simply observing the patient. Examples include ptosis, proptosis, Bell's palsy, extent of trauma (lacerations, edema, etc.).
- The slit lamp, which is usually performed by an ophthalmologist.
- Funduscopic exam, preferably with dilation of the pupil.

MANAGEMENT OF THE GERIATRIC PATIENT WITH VISION LOSS

Visual complaints should be addressed promptly by an ophthalmologist. General management for elderly patients consist of ensuring adequate lighting in the home, use of visual aids (e.g., large-print publications), and home safety evaluations for patients at risk of falling. Hospitalized patients should have access to corrective eyewear to help prevent delirium (see Chap. 4, Delirium).

OCULAR PATHOLOGY

Ocular pathology is more common in the geriatric population. Whereas glaucoma and age-related macular degeneration (ARMD) are not confined to the geriatric population, the incidence of these disorders increases with age. Although both of these conditions are progressive and can result in debilitating vision loss, treatment is available, and therefore all geriatric patients should be routinely screened for their presence.

Glaucoma

Glaucoma is a condition of progressive optic nerve damage usually related to increased intraocular pressure (IOP) (low-tension glaucoma is typically a disease of the young but may manifest in older patients). IOP >21 mm Hg is considered ocular HTN. If there is evidence of visual field loss or optic nerve fiber degeneration (progres-

TABLE 19-1. MEDICATIONS USED FOR THE TREATMENT OF GLAUCOMA

Medication	Examples	Indications/ contraindications	Mechanism of action	Ocular side effects	Systemic side effects
Beta blockers	Timolol Levobunolol-Metipranolol Betaxolol[b]	First-line therapy. Do not use in patients in whom systemic beta blockers would be contraindicated.	Decrease aqueous production[a]	Minimal	Same as for systemic beta blockers, including bradycardia, bronchospasm, fatigue, depression, exercise intolerance
Prostaglandin inhibitors	Latanoprost (Xalatan) Bimatoprost (Lumigan) Travoprost (Travatan)	Need for >6-mm decrease in intraocular pressure after beta blocker. Not yet approved as first-line agent, but is routinely used clinically as first-line agent for its greater efficacy.	Increase uveal scleral outflow[a]	Conjunctival hyperemia, hypertrichiasis, iris hyperchromia, ocular inflammation, macular edema	Minimal
Topical carbonic anhydrase inhibitors	Dorzolamide Brinzolamide	Second-line agent to be used when a single agent is not effective; contraindicated in persons with sulfa allergy.	Decrease aqueous production	Drop is viscous, and irritation is frequently a reason for discontinuation	Minimal
Alpha$_2$-adrenergic agonists	Apraclonidine Brimonidine	Second-line agent useful in patients who cannot tolerate beta blockers.	Decrease aqueous production	High rate of allergic reaction (up to 30%)	CNS side effects include lethargy

(continued)

TABLE 19-1. CONTINUED

Medication	Examples	Indications/ contraindications	Mechanism of action	Ocular side effects	Systemic side effects
Systemic carbonic anhydrase inhibitors	Acetazolamide Methazolamide	Useful for uncontrolled ocular HTN, usually short-term use, rarely for long-term use in nonsurgical candidates; contraindicated in persons with sulfa allergy, preexisting acidosis, sickle cell disease or trait.	Decrease aqueous production	Minimal	Induces systemic acidosis; causes metallic taste in mouth and tingling in fingers and toes
Hyperosmotic agents	Mannitol Glycerin Isosorbide	Useful short-term in uncontrolled ocular HTN.	Decrease vitreous hydration and volume	Minimal	Glycerin can cause hyperglycemia in diabetic patients, can induce heart failure due to increased vascular volume

[a]Mechanism unknown.
[b]Relatively cardioselective with fewer pulmonary side effects.

sive "cupping") associated with increased IOP, a patient has glaucoma. For patients with advanced glaucoma, there is good evidence that pressures <12 mm Hg need to be achieved to minimize the risk of progressive visual field loss. In patients with mild to moderate loss, the goal is to maintain a pressure at which there is no progression of visual field loss or cupping. **Treatment involves lowering IOP pharmacologically or surgically.** The goal of IOP varies by patient. The mainstay of treatment is a topical antihypertensive agent (Table 19-1). There are a number of different classes of drugs, but the most commonly prescribed drops act by two main mechanisms: to decrease aqueous humor production or to increase uveal-scleral outflow of aqueous. In acute glaucoma, PO carbonic anhydrase inhibitors can be given [acetazolamide (Diamox)], but there are significant side effects associated with these medications, and they are rarely used as maintenance therapy.

For patients who have failed medications or who are noncompliant with medication, there are a number of surgical approaches to mechanically increase the outflow of aqueous humor. The first is **laser trabeculoplasty.** A laser is used to "open" drainage canals within the trabecular meshwork when only a modest reduction in IOP is necessary. **"Filtering" surgery** is the most common procedure for attaining significant decreases in IOP. These procedures "bypass" the trabecular meshwork drainage by creating a direct pathway from the anterior chamber to the subconjunctival space. Although these procedures are the most likely to give a substantial decrease in IOP, they are not without short-term and long-term risks. The eye can become hypotonus (pathologically low pressure) immediately after filtering surgery or at any time postop if the filter begins to leak. These patients are at an increased risk of endophthalmitis (intraocular infection) because of the direct communication of the anterior chamber with the conjunctiva.

Age-Related Macular Degeneration

ARMD is a neurodegenerative disease that primarily affects the retinal pigment epithelium. Once the retinal pigment epithelium is damaged, however, photoreceptors in that area of the retina cannot be supported, and they also degenerate. ARMD represents the leading cause of irreversible vision loss in the elderly. There are two basic forms: the dry or atrophic form and the wet or exudative form. ARMD should be monitored by an ophthalmologist, and the patient should follow his or her own progress using an Amsler grid at home to pick up any sudden changes in visual function. **The dry form is slowly progressive and leads to decreased central visual acuity but rarely results in the severe vision loss that is associated with the wet form.** There is no effective therapy for the dry form of ARMD.

In **the wet or exudative form of ARMD,** patients develop subretinal neovascular membranes that are prone to leakage and/or hemorrhage. It is the damage created by these membranes that leads to devastating vision loss. The neovascular membranes can sometimes be treated either directly with thermal laser therapy or using photosensitive dye and an infrared laser (photodynamic therapy). Others may be removed surgically. Although therapies do exist, the prognosis for patients with ARMD and a neovascular membrane is generally poor. Zinc and antioxidants may have a role in slowing the progression of ARMD [2].

KEY POINTS TO REMEMBER

- Vision impairment contributes to functional decline, falls, delirium, and motor vehicle collisions.
- Ocular pathology is common in the elderly. Aging is associated with dry eyes, presbyopia, cataracts, "floaters," glaucoma, and macular degeneration.
- Biannual eye exam for screening elderly patients with no visual complaints is recommended as part of a health maintenance plan.
- Glaucoma treatment may consist of medications or surgery. Topical agents may have systemic side effects.
- ARMD is the leading cause of permanent vision loss in the elderly.

SUGGESTED READING

Abyad A. In-office screening for age-related hearing and vision loss. *Geriatrics* 1997; 52:45–57.

Butler RN, Faye EE, Guazzo E, et al. Keeping an eye on vision: primary care of age-related ocular disease. *Geriatrics* 1997;52:30–41.

Kalina RE. Aging and visual function. In: Hazzard WR, ed. *Principles of geriatric medicine and gerontology*, 4th ed. New York: McGraw-Hill, 1998.

McGwin G, Chapman V, Owsley C. Visual risk factors for driving difficulty among older drivers. *Accid Anal Prev* 2000;32:735–744.

REFERENCES

1. Owsley C, McGwin G, Sloane M, et al. Impact of cataract surgery on motor vehicle crash involvement by older adults. *JAMA* 2002;288:841–849.
2. Age-Related Eye Disease Study Research Group. A randomized, placebo-controlled clinical trial of high dose supplementation with vitamins C and E, beta-carotene, and zinc for age related macular degeneration and vision loss. *Arch Ophthalmol* 2001;119:1417–1436.

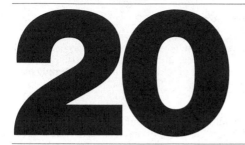

Aging and the Cardiovascular System, Exercise, and Hypertension

Roger Kerzner and
Rebecca M. Shepherd

AGING AND THE CARDIOVASCULAR SYSTEM

There are four clinically important areas of changes in the cardiovascular system that affect normal functioning and disease states. Changes in the kidneys, lungs, and neurohumoral system that occur with normal aging also contribute to the manifestations of cardiovascular disease in the elderly.

Increased Vascular Stiffness

The distensibility of large and medium-sized arteries decreases as the vessel walls become thicker with less elastin and more collagen. This stiffness is a component of aging and not accounted for by the increased prevalence of atherosclerotic disease. This manifests as systolic HTN and subsequent risk for coronary heart disease, heart failure, and stroke.

Impaired Ventricular Filling

A combination of an increase in collagen deposition, myocyte hypertrophy, and altered calcium mechanics contributes to impaired ventricular relaxation and decreased ventricular compliance. This manifests as diastolic dysfunction. The atrial component of ventricular filling becomes more important and magnifies the negative effects of atrial fibrillation. Also, the Frank-Starling mechanism to enhance stroke volume is diminished.

Reduced Ability to Increase Cardiac Output during Exercise or Stress

Both the ability to augment ATP production and respond to beta-adrenergic stimulation decline with aging.

Degeneration of the Conduction System

Impaired function of the sinus node and atrial conduction system predisposes elderly patients to brady- and tachyarrhythmias, especially atrial fibrillation.

EXERCISE IN THE ELDERLY

Aging is associated with a more sedentary lifestyle that is a risk factor for cardiovascular disease. Increasing fitness and participation in a regular program of physical activity can reduce the cardiovascular risk and diminish the effects of aging in relation to functional decline and adverse health [1]. Specifically, **exercise has been associated with improved longevity, body composition and strength, fewer falls, reduced depression, less arthritis pain, and lower risk for diabetes and coronary artery disease** [2].

Methods for Increasing Physical Activity in the Elderly

Lifestyle Modification

As many elderly persons are sedentary, the first goal may be to incorporate more activity into a patient's daily routine [1]. This can include parking farther away at stores or malls, climbing a flight of stairs instead of taking an elevator, or simply placing one's chair farther away from the kitchen.

Resistance Training

Exercises incorporating lifting of free weights or using commercially available equipment have the most impact in improving muscle strength and balance. Older persons should be counseled to avoid the Valsalva maneuver, as it can lead to decreased venous return to the right heart and hypotension.

Aerobic Exercise

In patients who are already generally active, aerobic exercise should be recommended for cardiopulmonary fitness. Exercises to consider include brisk walking, cycling on a stationary bicycle, swimming, and water aquatics. A safe place to start is with low-intensity exercise, as perceived by the patient. This can be gradually increased over weeks to months to a moderate level as tolerated.

For patients who have experienced myocardial infarction or had cardiac surgery, cardiac rehabilitation programs are equally effective in younger and older persons and are recommended [3].

Exercise Prescription

Formally writing a prescription for exercise can reinforce the importance of physical activity. It should be individualized and take into consideration the patient's interests, financial restraints, and comorbid medical conditions that may limit certain activities. **Include specific information on the type of exercise, frequency, duration, and any symptoms that should lead to discontinuing the exercise and contacting the physician.**

HYPERTENSION IN THE ELDERLY

HTN is the main risk factor for coronary artery disease, heart failure, and stroke in the elderly. Detection of high BP is important, as it is a treatable cause of morbidity and mortality. The National Health and Nutrition Examination Survey (NHANES III [4]) defined HTN as SBP >140 mm Hg and DBP >90 mm Hg. Also discovered during NHANES III is the fact that **average SBP tends to rise in both men and women throughout life, whereas DBP peaks around age 55 yrs.**

Isolated systolic HTN is a disease of older adults defined as an average SBP >160 with a DBP <90 mm Hg. The Systolic Hypertension in the Elderly Program [5] from 1994 estimates prevalence at 5–10% in adults aged 60–80 yrs and >20% in those ≥ 80 yrs. Treatment of isolate systolic HTN is recommend to reduce the risk of stroke, coronary events, heart failure, and death.

Despite the high prevalence of HTN in the elderly, it should not be considered a normal part of aging. **HTN is an independent risk factor for cardiovascular events.** Older adults have twice as many cardiovascular events as younger adults. Large placebo-controlled studies examining systolic HTN and/or diastolic HTN determined that treatment with antihypertensive therapy is beneficial to the older adult with high BP. Studies show that older adults treated with antihypertensive drugs have a 22% reduction in cardiovascular mortality, 15% reduction in coronary events, and 35% reduction in strokes.

Pathophysiology

HTN in the elderly may be physiologically different from that in younger adults in several ways. Older patients have less compliant blood vessels than younger patients owing to loss of elasticity and the presence of atherosclerosis. Decrease in beta-adrenergic responsiveness of smooth muscle impairs relaxation, and left ventricular mass is increased. Plasma renin levels change, as does renin responsiveness to orthostasis and volume depletion.

Secondary Hypertension

Secondary HTN is **unusual in the elderly population,** occurring in approximately 5% of cases. Secondary causes that are reasonable to consider in the older adult include renal artery stenosis, hypercalcemia, pheochromocytoma, and primary aldosteronism.

Secondary HTN should be considered in the following cases:

* **Drug-resistant HTN**
* **Previously well-controlled HTN** that is now difficult to control
* **Severe HTN** with diastolic pressures >115 mm Hg
* **Abnormal physical exam or lab data** suggestive of a secondary cause (abdominal bruit, hypokalemia, etc.)

History and Physical

HTN is usually **asymptomatic** and is found on routine BP measurement. On occasion, patients present with symptoms of hypertensive emergency with headache, encephalopathy, dizziness, blurred vision, chest pain, heart failure, or hematuria.

Accurate BP measurement is based on the average of two or more readings taken at each of two or more office visits. This is important in the elderly patients as their BP fluctuates more widely than a younger patient's does. **BP should be taken both sitting and supine, as elderly patients are more susceptible to postural hypotension** (see Chap. 8, Dizziness, Syncope, and Orthostatic Hypotension).

Erroneous elevation in HTN can occur because of decreased compliance and compressibility of atherosclerotic brachial arteries; this is called **pseudohypertension,** which can cause up to 15 mm Hg in error. There is no good way to overcome pseudohypertension other than intraarterial monitoring, which is not reasonable in the outpatient setting.

Examing for any involvement of **cardiovascular disease** is important, with attention to pulses, bruits (both carotid and renal), and evidence of left ventricular hypertrophy.

Management

Treatment of HTN in the elderly is indicated to reduce morbidity and mortality from cardiovascular and cerebrovascular events. **Recommended goals should be a DBP of ≤85–90 mm Hg in patients with diastolic HTN and a lowering of SBP of 20 mm Hg or a final SBP <160 mm Hg for those with systolic HTN.** In reducing BP in older patients, several special considerations must be made.

* In general, for antihypertensive drugs, **a lower initial dose is initiated than would be started in a younger patient** because of increased sensitivity to drug effects (including adverse effects).
* **BP should be reduced gradually** to minimize the risk of cerebral ischemia.
* The fragile elderly require even more caution when prescribing antihypertensive drugs or behavior modifications, as these patients have generally not been included in randomized controlled studies.
* Intervention with antihypertensive therapy has not been shown to affect patient mood or physical and mental abilities in general, **although patients with cerebral vascular disease may experience impaired cognitive function, depressed mood, and fatigue with standard BP reduction.** Serial cognitive evaluations on and off treatment may be warranted.

There is some evidence that **behavior modifications** reduce HTN. **Lifestyle modifications include the following:**

* Salt restriction
* Weight reduction
* Exercise
* High-fiber/reduced-fat diet
* Potassium supplementation
* Calcium supplementation
* Magnesium supplementation
* Fish oil supplementation

Antihypertensive drug treatment has been evaluated in numerous randomized, controlled trials and has been shown to decrease morbidity and mortality overall from cardiovascular events. These trials generally have examined the benefits of beta blockers and diuretics and focus on patients aged 60–80 yrs. **First-line therapy includes thiazide diuretics.** Trials as discussed earlier show improved morbidity and mortality. They also improve medical compliance with once-daily dosing and low cost. **Approximately 65% of older adults with HTN can be successfully treated with diuretics as the single agent.** Low-dose hydrochlorothiazide (12.5–25 mg PO qd) generally allows for good BP control with a low risk of side effects, such as **hypokalemia and postural hypotension.** Some elderly women are particularly susceptible to hyponatremia after initiating thiazide diuretics. Avoid using for patients with hypercalcemia, gout, urinary frequency, incontinence, and nocturia.

Beta blockers are appropriate first agents and should be considered for patients with a higher risk of cardiovascular events. Beta blockers are effective at lowering SBP in older patients and also decrease fatal and nonfatal cardiovascular events. They may not have the efficacy that is seen in younger patients because of decreased myocardial beta-adrenergic responsiveness and low renin levels, thus blunting the beta-blocking effect on these systems. **A small dose should be initiated and increased if well tolerated.** Contraindications to using beta blockers in the older patient include cardiac conduction defects, uncompensated heart failure, reactive airways disease, severe peripheral vascular disease, and poorly controlled insulin-dependent diabetes mellitus. **Beta blockers may cause fatigue, somnolence, and depression** and should be used with caution in the older adult with neuropsychological disease. In these patients, the water-soluble beta blockers may have fewer neurologic effects. **If maximally dosed thiazides or beta blockers alone or in combination do not control BP,** another agent will be required.

* **ACE inhibitors may be considered first-line treatment for some groups of patients,** particularly those with proteinuria, diabetic nephropathy, diabetes mellitus, peripheral vascular disease, cerebral vascular disease, and congestive heart failure. Combinations of ACE inhibitors and diuretics may have complementary effects. The Heart Outcomes Prevention Evaluation trial [6] showed improved cardiovascular outcomes for patients treated with ramipril. ACE inhibitor administration should be followed closely for evidence of hyperkalemia, hypotension, decreased renal function, angioedema, and cough.
* **Calcium-channel blockers** (CCBs) have limited morbidity and mortality end points supporting their use in the elderly population. The Systolic Hypertension in Europe trial [7] demonstrated that long-acting dihydropyridine CCBs (amlodipine, nimodipine) reduce cardiovascular morbidity and mortality in elderly patients with HTN. Other studies have demonstrated an increased risk of cognitive impairment and cardiovascular disease as compared with ACE inhibitors. CCBs cause vasodilatation while maintaining coronary blood flow. They appear to have increased potency in older patients, so a lower dose should be started. Side effects that limit their use include conduction abnormalities, headache, sodium retention, and peripheral edema.
* **Clonidine** has a number of side effects such as somnolence, dry mouth, constipation, and depression that are not well tolerated in the elderly population. Rebound HTN occurs when clonidine is suddenly discontinued or doses are missed.
* **Hydralazine** (Apresoline) and **reserpine** (Serpalan; Serpasil) are generally avoided because of adverse effects.

- **Alpha blockers** can be used in the setting of prostatism and HTN, although postural hypotension is a significant side effect.
- **Nitrates** are useful in the setting of HTN and stable angina but can cause headache and hypotension in the older patient.

Follow-Up

Patients should have regular follow-up with their physician at least twice yearly to check BP control, orthostatics, symptomatic side effects, and effect on volume status and electrolytes.

KEY POINTS TO REMEMBER

- There are four clinically important areas of changes in the cardiovascular system that affect normal functioning and disease states: increased vascular stiffness, impaired ventricular filling and relaxation, reduced ability to increase cardiac output during exercise or stress, and degeneration of the conduction system.
- Improving fitness and participation in a regular program of physical activity can reduce the cardiovascular risk and diminish the effects of aging in relation to functional decline and adverse health outcomes.
- HTN is not a normal part of aging and continues to be a major risk factor for stroke, coronary events, heart failure, and mortality at all ages.
- Isolated systolic HTN is a disease of older adults defined as an average SBP >160 mm Hg with a diastolic pressure <90 mm Hg. Treatment reduces the risk of stroke, coronary events, heart failure, and death.
- First-line agents for the treatment of HTN in the elderly include diuretics, beta blockers, and ACE inhibitors. Behavior modifications should be instituted.

SUGGESTED READING

Applegate WB, Pressel S, Wittes J, et al. Impact of the treatment of isolated systolic hypertension on behavioral variable. Results from the Systolic Hypertension in the Elderly Program. *Arch Intern Med* 1994;154:2154.
Beard K, Bulpitt C, Mascie-Taylor H, et al. Management of elderly patients with diastolic hypertension. *BMJ* 1992;304:412.
Insua JT, Sacks HS, Lau TS, et al. Drug treatment of hypertension in the elderly: a meta-analysis. *Ann Intern Med* 1994;121:355.
Karre R, Ouslander J. Cardiovascular disorders. In: Kane RL, Ouslander JG, Abrass IB, eds. *Essentials of clinical geriatrics*, 4th ed. New York: McGraw-Hill, 1999:294–301.
Lakatta EG. Circulatory function in younger and older humans in health. In Hazzard WR, ed. *Principles of geriatric medicine and gerontology*, 4th ed. New York: McGraw-Hill, 1999:645–660.
Lever AF, Pamsay LE. Treatment of hypertension in the elderly. *J Hypertens* 1995;13:571.
Mulrow CD, Brand MB. Hypertension in the elderly. In: Gallo JJ, Busby-Whitehead J, et al., eds. *Reichel's care of the elderly: clinical aspects of aging*, 5th ed. Philadelphia: Lippincott Williams & Wilkins, 1999:129–140.
Schwartz RS, Buchner DM. Exercise in the elderly: physiologic and functional effects. In: Hazzard WR, editor. *Principles of geriatric medicine and gerontology*, 4th ed. New York: McGraw-Hill, 1999:143–158.
The sixth report of the Joint National Committee on prevention, detection, evaluation, and treatment of high blood pressure. *Arch Intern Med* 1997;157:2413–2446.

REFERENCES

1. Christmas C, Andersen RA. Exercise and older patients: guidelines for the clinician. *J Am Geriatr Soc* 2000;48:318–24.
2. American College of Sports Medicine Position Stand. Exercise and physical activity for older adults. *Med Sci Sports Exerc* 1998;14:992–1008.

3. Lavie CJ, Milani RV. Effects of cardiac rehabilitation programs on exercise capacity, coronary risk factors, behavioral characteristics, and quality of life in a large elderly cohort. *Am J Cardiol* 1995;76:177–179.
4. Burt VL, Whelton P, Rocecella EJ, et al. Prevalence of Hypertension in the US Adult Population. Results from the Third National Health and Nutrition Examination Survey, 1988–1991. *Hypertension* 1995;25:305–313.
5. Prevention of stroke by antihypertensive drug treatment in the older patients with isolated systolic hypertension. Final results of the Systolic Hypertension in the Elderly Program (SHEP). SHEP Cooperative Research Group. *JAMA* 1991;265:3255–3264.
6. Yusuf S, Sleight P, Pogue J, et al. Effects of an angiotensin-converting-enzyme inhibitor, ramipril, on cardiovascular events in high-risk patients: the Heart Outcomes Prevention Evaluation Study Investigators. *N Engl J Med* 2000;342:145–153.
7. Staessen JA, Fagard R, Thijs L, et al. Randomised double-blind comparison of placebo and active treatment in older patients with isolated systolic hypertension. The Systolic Hypertension in Europe (Syst-Eur) Trial Investigators. *Lancet* 1997;350:757.

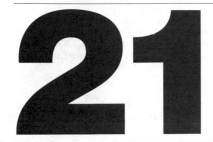

Ischemic Heart Disease

Roger Kerzner

CORONARY ARTERY DISEASE

Atherosclerosis is extremely common in elderly individuals, with a 70% prevalence by autopsy studies [1]. The severity of coronary artery lesions in men typically exceeds those in women until menopause, after which **men and women have nearly equal degrees of stenosis by their late 70s to early 80s.** These lesions tend to be diffuse, with three-vessel and left main coronary artery disease (CAD) being more common in elderly vs. younger patients. Subsequently, **85% of all deaths due to CAD occur in patients >65 yrs** [2].

Risk Factor Modification

Treating risk factors for CAD in older individuals can have a greater impact than similar treatments applied to younger patients. Whereas the relative risk of some factors declines with aging, the higher prevalence of CAD leads to a greater attributable risk. In other words, **the numbers of patients needed to treat for a specific risk factor to reduce cardiovascular events declines with aging.**

Hypertension

Numerous studies have demonstrated that treatment of elderly patients with hypertension reduces the incidence of CAD, heart failure, and stroke. (See Chap. 20, Aging and the Cardiovascular System, Exercise, and Hypertension).

Hyperlipidemia

Total and low-density lipoprotein cholesterol levels correlate with fatal CAD events, although the relative risk declines with aging [3]. **The ratio of total cholesterol to high-density lipoprotein cholesterol maintains its predictive power over the age of 75 yrs in both genders.**

In **patients with CAD,** subgroup analyses of patients >75 yrs in the three randomized controlled trials of therapy with HMG-CoA reductase inhibitors ("statins") for hyperlipidemia demonstrated a reduction in all-cause mortality and cardiovascular events. This was not accompanied by an increase in adverse events among elderly vs. younger patients. Thus, for secondary prevention of CAD in the elderly >75 yrs, therapy with an HMG-CoA reductase inhibitor in conjunction with a low-fat diet is recommended. Per the National Cholesterol Education Program III guidelines, the goals of therapy should be a low-density lipoprotein level <100 [4].

In **patients without CAD,** the screening and treatment of elevated cholesterol levels in patients >65 yrs have not been adequately studied. It may be reasonable to treat these patients if they do not have other comorbidities that could limit their lifespan. This should at least include dietary modifications and exercise. If drug therapy is selected, an HMG-CoA reductase inhibitor is the preferred treatment and may have other potential benefits for stroke reduction and treatment of dementia and osteoporosis [5–7].

Smoking
Tobacco abuse has been confirmed as a cardiovascular risk factor in older men and women [8]. **Cessation of smoking reduces the risk, even in individuals >70 yrs** [9]. Consider the use of smoking cessation programs, nicotine replacement therapy, or bupropion.

Diabetes
Diabetes remains a risk factor for CAD in the elderly. However, the cardiovascular benefits of aggressive treatment of diabetes in elderly patients are unknown.

Exercise
See Chap. 20, Aging and the Cardiovascular System, Exercise, and Hypertension.

ACUTE MYOCARDIAL INFARCTION AND UNSTABLE ANGINA

The incidence of acute myocardial infarctions (MIs) increases with age, along with rates of in-hospital mortality, arrhythmias, mechanical complications, and length of stay [10]. Unlike younger patients, an **equal number of men and women experience MIs after the age of 65 yrs, and it is the leading cause of death in this age group.** The type of MI also shifts toward **>50% being non–ST-segment elevation MIs.** These do not carry a benign prognosis in older persons, as **they are at increased risk for reinfarction, heart failure, and death** [11]. The incidence of silent or unrecognized MIs also increases with age (Table 21-1).

TABLE 21-1. ACUTE MYOCARDIAL INFARCTION (MI) AND UNSTABLE ANGINA IN THE ELDERLY

Clinical features	Relative frequency in older vs. younger patients
Epidemiology:	
Number of MIs	Increased
Number of silent or unrecognized MIs	Increased
Numbers of MIs; men vs. women	1:1
Numbers of MIs; ST-segment elevation vs. non–ST-segment elevation	1:1
Rate of in-hospital mortality, length of stay, arrhythmias and mechanical complications	Increased
Risk of reinfarction and heart failure	Increased
Risk of death from acute MI	Increased
Presenting symptom:	
Dyspnea	Increased
Chest pain	Decreased
Diaphoresis	Decreased
Dizziness, confusion, syncope	Increased
Physical exam and ECG:	
Variability of exam; normal vs. abnormal	Increased
Pulmonary edema	Increased
Nondiagnostic ECG	Increased

Presentation

History

The rule in older persons with MIs is that they present with atypical symptoms [11]. The most common complaint after the age of 75 yrs is **dyspnea.** Chest pain and diaphoresis are less common than in younger individuals, whereas nonspecific neurologic symptoms such as **dizziness, confusion, and syncope may be the presenting symptoms in 20% of patients >85 yrs.** Symptoms as seemingly unrelated as stroke, vertigo, weakness, abdominal pain, nausea, vomiting, and cough may be secondary to an acute coronary syndrome. Thus, a high index of suspicion for an MI is essential when evaluating an older man or woman with an acute illness.

Physical Exam

The physical exam is also variable in the elderly. Patients can have a normal or abnormal temperature, respiratory rate, heart rate, and heart rhythm. They may appear ill or comfortable. Despite its lack of use in diagnosis, the exam is important in assessing hemodynamic status and looking for pulmonary edema, which is more commonly associated with MIs in the elderly. Up to 40% of older patients with an acute MI have heart failure [11].

Diagnostic Evaluation

An **ECG** should be performed on all patients with a suspected acute coronary syndrome, although it is often nondiagnostic in older patients. This results from preexisting ECG abnormalities (e.g., left ventricular hypertrophy, left bundle branch block, or paced rhythms) and the higher prevalence of non–ST-elevation MIs. Serum markers of myocardial damage (i.e., troponin-I) are thus an integral part of the diagnostic evaluation.

Management

Reperfusion Therapy

If an acute MI is diagnosed, consideration must be given to reperfusion therapy. **Older age is not a contraindication to thrombolysis or angioplasty, and these therapies may have a greater absolute impact in elderly patients** [12]

FIBRINOLYTIC THERAPY. Pooled analysis from five large, randomized, placebo-controlled trials of thrombolytic therapy administered within 6 hrs of symptom onset in elderly patients with an acute ST-segment elevation MI indicated a significant reduction in mortality [13]. **Although the risk of intracranial hemorrhage increases with age, the total mortality benefit still exists.**

CORONARY ANGIOPLASTY. Primary percutaneous transluminal coronary angioplasty (PTCA) may be the preferred reperfusion strategy in elderly patients presenting to experienced centers that can perform the procedure within 90 mins of a patient's arrival in the ER. This was demonstrated in the Global Use of Strategies to Open Occluded Coronary Arteries in Acute Coronary Syndromes (GUSTO IIb) trial comparing PTCA with rt-PA, in which 300 patients >70 yrs had an improved composite end point of death, reinfarction, or disabling stoke [14]. Less information is known about primary PTCA in patients >80 yrs [15].

In the setting of non–ST-segment elevation MIs, an early invasive strategy is also indicated in selected patients >65 yrs. The TACTICS-TIMI 18 (Treat Angina with Aggrastat and Determine Cost of Therapy with an Invasive or Conservative Strategy–Thrombolysis in Myocardial Infarction 18 Investigators) trial demonstrated that intermediate- and high-risk patients treated with PTCA within 48 hrs and early administration of a glycoprotein IIb/IIIa inhibitor had a reduced combined end point of death, nonfatal MI, or rehospitalization for an acute coronary syndrome at 6 mos [16]. The role of this strategy in patients >75 yrs is unclear because of limited data.

One subgroup of patients who should not undergo primary PTCA is patients >75 yrs with an acute MI complicated by cardiogenic shock. These patients benefit more from initial medical stabilization with thrombolytics and intraaortic balloon counterpulsation as necessary [17].

TABLE 21-2. MEDICATIONS USED FOR ACUTE MYOCARDIAL INFARCTION (MI) OR UNSTABLE ANGINA

Medication	Comments [reference]
ASA, 160–325 mg PO	Absolute mortality benefit of ASA increases from 1% in patients younger than 60 to 4.7% in those ≥ 70 yrs [12].
Other antiplatelet agents	Appropriate use unclear in elderly patients.
	There is no specific contraindication to the use of IIb/IIIa inhibitors in regards to aging [34], but dosing for the patient's renal function should be used.
Heparin	
Unfractionated	Unproven value. A recent retrospective chart review of patients >65 yrs hospitalized with acute MI demonstrated more bleeding complications without reduction in mortality or reinfarction in patients treated with unfractionated heparin [35].
Low-molecular-weight heparin	May be preferred agent in elderly [36].
Beta blockers	Elderly patients derive a 23% reduction in mortality with early IV beta blockers.
	Lower doses may be appropriate in older patients.
ACE inhibitors	Early treatment within 24 hrs after MI reduces mortality and heart failure in patients >70 yrs [37–39].
	Start with a low dose of a short-acting ACE inhibitor (captopril, 6.25 mg PO q6–8h), and gradually increase the dose as tolerated.
	The risk of renal dysfunction and hypotension is greater in older patients and should be continually monitored.
	IV enalaprilat should not be used, as it can cause serious hypotension in patients >70 yrs [24].
Nitrates	Safe in most elderly patients.
	Favorable trends in mortality seen in patients >70 yrs [37].
Morphine	Can relieve pain and dyspnea but risk of delirium.
Antiarrhythmic agents	No benefit with routine use.
Blood transfusions	Observational data support the use of blood transfusions to maintain a Hct >30% in patients ≥ 65 yrs who have experienced an acute MI [40].

Medical Management
The agents listed in Table 21-2 are applicable to all elderly patients with acute MI or unstable angina.

CHRONIC CORONARY ARTERY DISEASE

As mentioned earlier, CAD is extremely common in elderly individuals and in many is a chronic problem. **With increasingly sedentary lifestyles, older patients tend to be asymptomatic or minimally symptomatic despite having more severe CAD.** This requires a high clinical index of suspicion for CAD and subsequent evaluation.

In older patients with their first manifestation of CAD, unstable angina is the most common presentation [18]. Younger patients more commonly sustain acute MI as their initial manifestation and, less commonly, heart failure or sudden death.

Management

Diagnosis

The same principles regarding the symptoms and diagnosis of acute MIs in older persons apply to chronic CAD. Atypical presentations and nondiagnostic physical exams and ECGs often necessitate objective testing to certify the diagnosis of CAD and ensure appropriate treatment.

STRESS TESTING. The efficacy of all commonly used methods of stress testing for diagnosing CAD and predicting cardiac events in elderly patients has been demonstrated [19,20]. This includes ECG, either alone or in combination with radionuclide or echocardiographic imaging. **ECG alone may be limited in older persons because of baseline ECG abnormalities.**

In patients who can exercise to increase their heart rate to at least 80% of their predicted maximum, exercise testing is preferred over pharmacologic stress testing. Advanced age is not a contraindication for exercise testing and should be offered to most patients. For many patients who cannot exercise to an adequate level because of lack of physical fitness or comorbid medical conditions, dipyridamole, adenosine, and dobutamine are acceptable alternatives as pharmacologic stress testing agents.

Of the available methods of stress testing, aside from the benefits of exercise vs. a pharmacologic stress, none has uniformly improved accuracy in elderly patients. Considering the variability in the performance of these tests at different labs, a prudent approach is to choose the most trusted test at a particular institution [21].

DIAGNOSTIC CATHETERIZATION. Diagnostic catheterization can be safely performed in elderly patients but should be reserved for patients who will consider a revascularization procedure.

Medical Management

The pharmacologic treatment of chronic CAD is very similar in younger and older patients. It includes the use of ASA, beta blockers, ACE inhibitors, nitrates, calcium channel blockers, and risk factor modification. **The unique aspects in elderly patients predominantly relate to side effects associated with many of these medications.**

BETA BLOCKERS. Elderly individuals are more susceptible to fatigue, dizziness, depression, exercise intolerance, atrioventricular blockade, and impotence that can result from beta blockade. It may be necessary to reduce the dose of a patient's medication because of one of these side effects. Discontinuation of a beta blocker should be avoided if possible because of the substantial reduction in mortality in elderly patients, especially if they have suffered an MI [22]. This benefit persists in patients >65 yrs with left ventricular dysfunction who are also on an ACE inhibitor [23].

ACE INHIBITORS. ACE inhibitors are very safe medications in elderly patients. In patients who have experienced an MI complicated by heart failure or left ventricular dysfunction, long-term ACE inhibitor therapy reduces mortality, hospitalizations, and heart failure at least, if not more, effectively in older persons [24,25]. The decline in renal function associated with aging should not dissuade physicians from using ACE inhibitors.

CALCIUM CHANNEL BLOCKERS. Calcium channel blockers have **no beneficial effect on survival in patients with chronic CAD.** They can be useful antianginal agents but should only be used in patients who do not have relief of their symptoms with beta blockers and nitrates. Common side effects include **edema and constipation,** which may be particularly pronounced in elderly patients. The combination of beta blockers and calcium channel blockers may predispose to postural hypotension and atrioventricular blockade and should be used with caution.

Revascularization

PTCA and coronary artery bypass graft (CABG) operations are commonly performed in elderly patients to relieve symptoms, enhance quality of life, and potentially improve survival. **Currently, >50% of all PTCA and CABG procedures occur in patients >65 yrs,** and the proportion continues to rise [2]. However, information from randomized trials addressing the appropriate use of these procedures in elderly patients is minimal, especially for patients >75 yrs. Thus, the decision to pursue revascularization should incorporate the patient's wishes regarding the acute risks and long-term benefits of revascularization. Based on the available evidence, there are a few points to consider while making this difficult decision.

PERIOPERATIVE OUTCOMES. **The short-term mortality of PTCA and CABG increases with age** but has been declining over the last decade [26]. The in-hospital mortality rate of PTCA increases from <1% in 60-yr-old patients to 2–4% in octogenarians. With CABG, the risk is 2–3% in patients ≤ 60 yrs and rises to 5–8% after the age of 80 yrs. These higher mortality rates should be understood within the context of elderly vs. younger patients referred for either PTCA or CABG. **The older patients generally have more advanced CAD, more symptoms, and more comorbidities** [26,27], thus diluting the impact on mortality attributable to revascularization.

Beyond mortality, **postprocedural complications are higher after CABG vs. PTCA in older persons.** Approximately 3–6% of patients >75 yrs have a permanently disabling stoke or coma after CABG, as compared to <1% of after PTCA [26]. Other complications include atrial fibrillation, heart failure, bleeding, cognitive dysfunction, respiratory dysfunction, and renal insufficiency. The best predictor of complications is a patient's entire risk profile, including associated medical diseases and left ventricular function, rather than age alone [26,27].

SYMPTOM RELIEF. Relief of anginal symptoms refractory to medical therapy is a frequent and widely accepted indication for revascularization in the elderly. In comparison to younger patients, limited data suggest that **older patients experience equal or greater symptom relief and quality of life improvement after CABG** [26–28]. This is less clear in patients who undergo PTCA, mainly secondary to incomplete revascularization. In the "oldest old," PTCA may still be the best option for symptom relief because of the higher short-term risks of surgery.

LONG-TERM OUTCOMES. After the initial postop period, both revascularization procedures lead to improved quality of life in older patients vs. medical therapy alone [26,28,29]. Among octogenarians, 89% were found to be living independently 1 yr after CABG or PTCA, compared with 52% of those treated medically [30]. One observational study among elderly patients with multivessel CAD even showed significantly higher 7-yr survival rates in patients who underwent PTCA or CABG compared to those treated medically [31]. These data are subject to a selection bias, because patients treated medically are often not candidates for a revascularization procedure.

In comparing the two procedures, the available information from observational studies and registries on long-term morbidity outcomes appear to favor surgery. CABG has conferred greater improvements in functional outcomes, and PTCA is hindered by higher rates of repeat revascularization [26,27]. One registry found that in elderly patients with severe symptoms, CABG was also associated with better survival [32]. These benefits of CABG are counterbalanced by the long-term cognitive decline after surgery, which may persist in up to 42% of patients after 5 yrs [33].

UNKNOWN VARIABLES. The paucity of clinical trials on revascularization in elderly patients makes it difficult to judge whether the acute risks are outweighed by potential long-term benefits. Even less is known about which subgroups derive the most benefit from revascularization or how to assess functional outcomes or quality of life. The impact of technical improvements such as intracoronary stents and minimally invasive surgery is also unclear.

KEY POINTS TO REMEMBER

- With aging, fewer patients need to be treated for a specific CAD risk factor to achieve benefit.
- The incidence of acute MI increases with age.
- The type of MI changes as >50% are non–ST-segment elevation MIs. These do not carry a benign prognosis in older persons, as they are at increased risk for reinfarction, heart failure, and death.

- Older persons with acute MI usually present with atypical symptoms (e.g. dizziness, confusion, syncope).
- Older age is not a contraindication to thrombolysis or angioplasty, which have a greater absolute impact in elderly patients with acute MI.
- With increasingly sedentary lifestyles, older patients tend to be asymptomatic or minimally symptomatic despite having more severe CAD. This requires a high clinical index of suspicion for CAD and subsequent evaluation.
- The paucity of clinical trials on revascularization (PTCA and CABG) in elderly patients with chronic CAD makes it difficult to judge whether the acute risks are outweighed by potential long-term benefits.

SUGGESTED READING

Boden WE, O'Rourke RA, Crawford MH, et al. Outcomes in patients with acute non-Q-wave myocardial infarction randomly assigned to an invasive as compared with a conservative management strategy. *N Engl J Med* 1998;338:1785–1792.

GUSTO Investigators. An international randomized trial comparing four thrombolytic strategies for acute myocardial infarction. *N Engl J Med* 1993;329:673–682.

Kjoller-Hansen L, Steffensen R, Grande P. The angiotensin-converting enzyme inhibitor post revascularization study (APRES). *J Am Coll Cardiol* 2000;35:881–888.

Rich MW. Heart disease in the elderly. In: Rosendorff C, ed. *Essential cardiology: principles and practice*. Philadelphia: WB Saunders, 2001:722–743.

Rich MW. Therapy for acute myocardial infarction. *Clin Geriatr Med* 1996;12:121–168.

TIMI IIIB Investigators. Effects of tissue plasminogen activator and a comparison of early invasive and conservative strategies in unstable angina and non-Q wave myocardial infarction. Results of the TIMI IIIB trial. *Circulation* 1994;89:1545–1556.

REFERENCES

1. Aronow WS, Tresch DD. Recognition and diagnosis of coronary artery disease in the elderly. In: Tresch DD, Aronow WS, eds. *Cardiovascular disease in the elderly patient*, 2nd ed. New York: Marcel Dekker, 1999:197–212.
2. 2001 Heart and stroke biostatistical fact sheet. Dallas: American Heart Association, 2001. Available at: http://www.americanheart.org. Accessed May 2003.
3. Grundy SM, Cleeman JI, Rifkind BM, et al. Cholesterol lowering in the elderly population. *Arch Intern Med* 1999;159:1670–1678.
4. Executive Summary of The Third Report of The National Cholesterol Education Program (NCEP) Expert Panel on Detection, Evaluation, And Treatment of High Blood Cholesterol In Adults (Adult Treatment Panel III). *JAMA* 2001;285(19):2486–2497.
5. Byington RP, Jukema JW, Salonen JT, et al. Reduction in cardiovascular events during pravastatin therapy. Pooled analysis of clinical events of the pravastatin atherosclerosis intervention program. *Circulation* 1995;92:2419–2425.
6. Jick H, Zornberg GL, Jick SS, et al. Statins and the risk of dementia. *Lancet* 2000;356(9242):1627–1631.
7. Meier CR, Schlienger RG, Kraenzlin ME, et al. HMG-CoA reductase inhibitors and the risk of fractures. *JAMA* 2000;283:3205–3210.
8. LaCroix AZ, Lang J, Scherr P, et al. Smoking and mortality among older men and women in three communities. *N Engl J Med* 1991;324:619–625.
9. Hermanson B, Omenn GS, Kronmal RA, et al. Beneficial six-year outcome of smoking cessation in older men and women with coronary artery disease. *N Engl J Med* 1988;319:1365–1369.
10. Wei JY. Coronary heart disease. In: Hazzard WR, ed. *Principles of geriatric medicine and gerontology*, 4th ed. New York: McGraw-Hill, 1999:661–668.
11. Tresch DD. Management of the older patient with acute myocardial infarction: Differences in clinical presentations between older and younger patients. *J Am Geriatr Soc* 1998;46:1157–1162.

12. ISIS-2 (Second International Study of Infarct Survival) Collaborative Group. Randomized trial of intravenous streptokinase, oral aspirin, both, or neither among 17187 cases of suspected acute myocardial infarction: ISIS-2. *Lancet* 1988;II:349–360.

13. Rich MW. Therapy for acute myocardial infarction in older persons. *J Am Geriatr Soc* 1998;46:1302–1307.

14. The Global Use of Strategies to Open Occluded Coronary Arteries in Acute Coronary Syndromes (GUSTO IIb) Angioplasty Substudy Investigators. A clinical trial comparing primary coronary angioplasty with tissue plasminogen activator for acute myocardial infarction. *N Engl J Med* 1997;336:1621–1628.

15. Laster SB, Rutherford BD, Giorgi LV, et al. Results of direct percutaneous transluminal coronary angioplasty in octogenarians. *Am J Cardiol* 1996;77:10–13.

16. Cannon CP, Weintraub WS, Demopoulos LA, et al. for the TACTICS-Thrombolysis in Myocardial Infarction 18 Investigators. Comparison of early invasive and conservative strategies in patients with unstable coronary syndromes treated with the glycoprotein IIb/IIIa inhibitor tirofiban. *N Engl J Med* 2001;344:1879–1887.

17. Hochman JS, Sleeper LA, Webb JG, et al. Early revascularization in acute myocardial infarction complicated by cardiogenic shock. *N Engl J Med* 1999;341:625–634.

18. Tresch DD, Saeian K, Hoffman R. Elderly patients with late onset of coronary artery disease: clinical and angiographic findings. *Am J Geriatr Cardiol* 1992;1:14–25.

19. Schulman SP, Fleg JL. Stress testing for coronary artery disease in the elderly. *Clin Geriatr Med* 1996;12:101–119.

20. Arruda AM, Das MK, Roger VL, et al. Prognostic value of exercise echocardiography in 2.632 patients >65 years of age. *J Am Coll Cardiol* 2001;37:1036–1041.

21. Lee TH, Boucher CA. Noninvasive tests in patients with stable coronary artery disease. *N Engl J Med* 2001;344:1840–1845.

22. Aronow WS. Management of older persons after myocardial infarction. *J Am Geriatr Soc* 1998;46:1459–1468.

23. Shlipak MG, Browner WS, Noguchi H, et al. Comparison of the effects of angiotensin converting-enzyme inhibitors and beta blockers on survival in elderly patients with reduced left ventricular function after myocardial infarction. *Am J Med* 2001;110:425–433.

24. Swedburg K, Held P, Kjekshus J, et al. Effects of early administration of enalapril on mortality in patients with acute myocardial infarction. Results of the Cooperative New Scandinavian Enalapril Survival Study (CONSENSUS II). *N Engl J Med* 1992;327:678–684.

25. The Acute Infarction Ramipril Efficacy (AIRE) Study Investigators. Effect of ramipril on mortality and morbidity of survivors of acute myocardial infarction with clinical evidence of heart failure. *Lancet* 1993;342:821–828.

26. Shapira I, Pines A, Mohr R. Updated review of the coronary artery bypass grafting option in octogenarians: good tidings. *Am J Geriatr Cardiol* 2001;10:199–206.

27. Singh M, Thompson RC, Holmes DR. Percutaneous transluminal coronary angioplasty in the elderly. In: Tresch DD, Aronow WS, eds. *Cardiovascular disease in the elderly patient*, 2nd ed. New York: Marcel Dekker, 1999:317–331.

28. The TIME Investigators. Trial of Invasive Versus Medical Therapy in Elderly Patients with Chronic Symptomatic Coronary-Artery Disease (TIME): a randomised trial. *Lancet* 2001;358:951–957.

29. Stemmer EA, Aronow WS. Surgical treatment of coronary artery disease in the elderly. In: Tresch DD, Aronow WS, eds. *Cardiovascular disease in the elderly patient*, 2nd ed. New York: Marcel Dekker, 1999:283–316.

30. Krumholz HM, Forman DE, Kuntz RE, et al. Coronary revascularization after myocardial infarction in the very elderly: outcomes and long term follow-up. *Ann Intern Med* 1993;119:1084–1090.

31. Peterson ED, Buell H, DeLong ER, et al. Do the very aged benefit from revascularization? Results from 2,613 pts aged 75 yrs in the Duke Database. *Circulation* 1999;100:1–84.

32. Gersh BJ, Kronmal RA, Schaff HV, et al. Comparison of coronary artery bypass surgery and medical therapy in patients 65 years of age and older. A nonrandomized study from the Coronary Artery Surgery Study (CASS) registry. *N Engl J Med* 1985;313:217–224.

33. Newman MF, Kirchner JL, Phillips-Bute B, et al. Longitudinal assessment of neurocognitive function after coronary-artery bypass surgery. *N Engl J Med* 2001;344:395–402.

34. Mak KH, Effron MB, Moliterno DJ. Platelet glycoprotein IIb/IIIa receptor antagonists and their use in elderly patients. *Drugs Aging* 2000;16:179–187.

35. Krumholz HM, Hennen J, Ridker PM, et al. Use and effectiveness of intravenous heparin therapy for treatment of acute myocardial infarction in the elderly. *J Am Coll Cardiol* 1998;31:973–979.

36. Cohen M, Demers C, Gurfinkel EP, et al. A comparison of low molecular weight heparin with unfractionated heparin for unstable coronary artery disease. *N Engl J Med* 1997;337:447–452.

37. GISSI-3: effects of lisinopril and transdermal glyceryl trinitrate singly and together on 6-week mortality and ventricular function after acute myocardial infarction. *Lancet* 1994;343:1115–1122.

38. Anbrosioni E, Borghi C, Magnani B. The effect of angiotensin-converting enzyme inhibitor zofenopril on mortality and morbidity after anterior myocardial infarction. *N Engl J Med* 1995;332:80–85.

39. Swedberg K, Held P, Kjekshus J, et al. Effects of the early administration of enalapril on mortality in patients with acute myocardial infarction. Results of the Cooperative New Scandinavian Enalapril Survival Study II (CONSENSUS II). *N Engl J Med* 1992;327:678–684.

40. Wen-Chih W, Rathore SS, Wang Y, et al. Blood transfusions in elderly patients with acute myocardial infarction. *N Engl J Med* 2001;345:1230–1236.

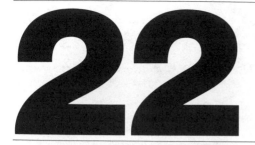

Chronic Heart Failure, Valvular Disease, and Arrhythmias

Roger Kerzner

CHRONIC HEART FAILURE

Heart failure is predominantly a geriatric syndrome that has become a major public health concern in the 21st century because of the aging population [1]. There are 550,000 new cases every year [1a]. It affects 10% of persons >80 yrs, whereas <1% of the population <50 yrs are affected [2]. Chronic heart failure (CHF) is the leading cause for hospitalization and rehospitalization in elderly individuals [3,4] and thus is the **most costly medical illness in the United States** [5].

Pathophysiology

The etiology for the increase in heart failure stems from a combination of the aging process (see Chap. 20, Aging and the Cardiovascular System, Exercise, and Hypertension) and comorbidities common in older persons. This includes increased vascular stiffness, impaired ventricular filling, diminished ATP production and response to neurohumoral stimuli, and degeneration of the conduction system. The end result is maintained cardiac performance at rest but diminished cardiac reserve. The impact of these factors is magnified by the high prevalence of systemic HTN and coronary artery disease. Stresses such as ischemia, tachycardia, systemic illness, or physical exertion, which are generally well tolerated in younger individuals, often lead to CHF in the elderly.

A distinguishing feature of heart failure in the elderly is the high prevalence of cases that occur in the setting of normal or near-normal left ventricular function (Table 22-1). This is commonly referred to as **diastolic dysfunction** or **diastolic heart failure.** It is the clinical result of the pathophysiology described earlier. Diastolic dysfunction accounts for >50% of heart failure in persons >75 yrs vs. <10% in those <65 yrs and is more common in women [6,7].

Clinical Features

History
Exertional dyspnea, orthopnea, lower extremity swelling, and **exercise intolerance** are the most common symptoms of CHF in older and younger persons (Table 22-1). However, with increasing age and often a more sedentary lifestyle, exertional symptoms become less common. Atypical and often nonspecific symptoms such as confusion, somnolence, irritability, fatigue, anorexia, nausea, and diminished activity level become more common. Subtle behavior changes to overt delirium often accompany CHF in elderly institutionalized or hospitalized patients [8].

As a result, **CHF is both overdiagnosed and underdiagnosed in the elderly.** Pulmonary or thyroid diseases, anemia, depression, or other primary CNS diseases can explain many of the symptoms described earlier. Particularly in the setting of an acute CHF exacerbation, clinicians should be wary of the multiple diagnostic possibilities that may lead to a patient's clinical scenario, rather than jumping to or ignoring the possibility of CHF.

TABLE 22-1. RELATIVE FREQUENCY OF CHRONIC HEART FAILURE FEATURES IN OLDER VS. YOUNGER PATIENTS

Clinical features	Relative frequency
Epidemiology	
Number of patients with chronic heart failure	Greatly increased
Percentage of patients with normal systolic function	Increased
Symptoms	
Exertional dyspnea	Decreased
Atypical and nonspecific symptoms (confusion, irritability, diminished activity)	Increased
Physical exam	
Elevated jugular venous pressure	Decreased
S3 gallop	Decreased
Pulmonary rales	Decreased
Peripheral edema	Decreased
Mental status changes	Increased

Physical Exam

As with symptoms, typical exam findings of elevated jugular venous pressure, an S3 gallop, pulmonary rales, and peripheral edema are less common in older patients with CHF (Table 22-1). It may be more important to pay attention to subtle mental status changes that may be the only finding of CHF. No single clinical feature can reliably determine whether heart failure is secondary to systolic or diastolic dysfunction; thus, an assessment of left ventricular function is essential.

Management

Diagnosis

A **chest x-ray** is a useful initial test in patients with suspected heart failure. Although it may be nondiagnostic in elderly individuals with mild symptoms, findings of cardiomegaly or pulmonary edema may confirm the diagnosis of CHF.

As no single clinical feature can reliably distinguish between a systolic or diastolic cause for heart failure, **an assessment of left ventricular function is essential.** This will affect treatment decisions (see Pharmacologic Management). **Echocardiography** is the least invasive and most widely used method and can provide additional information about chamber size and valvular lesions. Other diagnostic testing may be indicated to evaluate precipitating factors of CHF.

Precipitating Factors

In both the acute and chronic settings, **the multiple underlying causes and precipitating factors for each case of CHF should be investigated and treated appropriately.** HTN and coronary artery disease account for 70–80% of CHF cases at older age [9] and should be treated aggressively to improve symptoms (see Chap. 20, Aging and the Cardiovascular System, Exercise, and Hypertension, and Chap. 21, Ischemic Heart Disease). Other factors may particularly affect older patients.

    MEDICATION AND DIETARY COMPLIANCE. Multiple factors contribute to noncompliance with medical therapy in older persons. This is discussed in more detail in Nonpharmacologic Management.

    NSAIDS. NSAIDs are commonly used medications that promote salt and water retention, interfere with the actions of ACE inhibitors and other antihypertensive agents, and may worsen renal function, which can all contribute to heart failure. They must be used cautiously in elderly patients and be inquired about when patients are admitted for a CHF exacerbation. This is true for both nonselective and selective **COX-2 inhibitors.**

ALCOHOL. Alcoholism is common but often unrecognized in older persons. Alcohol use should be inquired about and strongly discouraged if an alcoholic cardiomyopathy is suspected.

ATRIAL FIBRILLATION. Atrial fibrillation (AF) is a common precipitant of heart failure in elderly patients, especially in those with diastolic dysfunction in whom the atrial component of diastolic filling of the left ventricle is more important. Ventricular rate control is essential at rest and during activity to maintain filling (see Atrial Fibrillation).

AORTIC STENOSIS. Severe aortic stenosis (AS) is more common in older persons and may be difficult to detect on exam. As older patients can be effectively treated with a valve replacement, the aortic valve should be evaluated in all older patients with heart failure (see Aortic Stenosis).

Pharmacologic Management
The first step in designing a treatment regimen is determining the presence of systolic dysfunction. Although diastolic dysfunction is likely present in all older patients with heart failure, proven therapies only exist for systolic dysfunction.

A particular caveat of treating elderly patients is frequent monitoring. Most of the medications discussed later can have significant effects on renal function and electrolytes, especially potassium. Routine lab testing of these indices should be obtained within 2 wks after a new medication is started or dose changed and periodically thereafter.

ACE INHIBITORS. These medications are the **first-line therapy** in patients with systolic dysfunction and continue to have benefits on mortality and quality of life in elderly patients [10,11]. Initiation of therapy should begin with a low dose (captopril [Capoten], 6.25–12.5 mg PO tid, or enalapril [Vasotec], 2.5 mg PO bid) and titrated slowly over many weeks. The goal should be doses effective in clinical trials (captopril, 50 mg tid; enalapril, 10 mg PO bid; and lisinopril [Prinivil, Zestril], 20 mg PO qd; ramipril [Altace], 5 mg PO bid; trandolapril [Mavik], 4 mg PO qd).

Close monitoring of renal function, electrolytes, and screening for orthostatic hypotension are essential, as older persons are more susceptible to these side effects. If necessary, the dosage can be reduced, as even low doses of an ACE inhibitor may be beneficial. Baseline renal insufficiency is not an absolute contraindication to a trial of an ACE inhibitor if renal function is monitored closely.

Angiotensin receptor blockers may have similar beneficial effects in older patients with heart failure but should be reserved for patients who are intolerant to ACE inhibitors until further clinical trials are completed.

BETA BLOCKERS. Decreased mortality and improved left ventricular function have been demonstrated in CHF patients up to the age of 80 yrs treated with beta blockers [12–14]. Treatment should be started only in stable patients already on an ACE inhibitor. The starting dose should be low (carvedilol [Coreg], 3.125 mg PO bid, or metoprolol [Lopressor, Toprol-XL], 6.25–12.5 mg PO bid) and titrated slowly over many weeks. This is especially true in older persons who have a higher prevalence of severe bradyarrhythmias and lung disease. Monitoring should include screening for fatigue, exercise intolerance, depression, and impotence, which may be side effects of beta blocker therapy.

DIURETICS. Relieving congestion and maintenance of euvolemia with diuretics are useful for maintaining the quality of life in patients with CHF. Thiazides, loop diuretics, and metolazone are all appropriate choices depending on the degree of volume overload. In older patients, it may be prudent to allow for a small degree of peripheral edema to prevent hypotension, which can result from overdiuresis. **As most older patients with CHF have a component of diastolic dysfunction, they are particularly sensitive to reductions in preload.**

Spironolactone (Aldactone) at a dose of 25 mg PO qd is indicated in patients with New York Heart Association class III-IV heart failure if severe renal insufficiency or hyperkalemia is not present [15].

DIGOXIN. Digoxin (Lanoxin) can improve symptoms and reduce hospitalizations in men but has no effect on mortality [16]. These benefits persist in patients >80 yrs. A dose of 0.125 mg PO qd provides a therapeutic effect in most older patients, but those at an estimated Cr clearance <50 should only take 0.125 mg every other day. If toxicity is suspected, a digoxin level can be measured with the therapeutic range being lowered to 0.5–1.3 ng/mL after the age of 70 yrs [17].

HYDRALAZINE AND NITRATES. The combination of hydralazine (Apresoline) and isosorbide dinitrate (Dilatrate-SR, Imdur, ISMO, Iso-Bid, Isordil, Isotrate, Sorbitrate) decreased mortality in a study of heart failure patients <75 yrs [18]. It has not been studied in older individuals but may be an effective alternative for afterload reduction in patients intolerant to ACE inhibitors.

Pharmacologic Management of Diastolic Dysfunction

To date, no large trials of a specific therapy for diastolic dysfunction have been completed. Pharmacologic management is empiric and should be guided by prevailing comorbidities and symptomatic relief. Ultimately, a trial of different medications may be the best way of managing pharmacotherapy in older patients with diastolic dysfunction.

Diuretics and nitrates can be used to relieve congestion and orthopnea, but cautious attention for overdiuresis and declining renal function is essential. Often seemingly minor increases in the dose of a diuretic can overwhelm the delicate volume status of older patients with diastolic dysfunction.

ACE inhibitors and beta blockers should be used in patients who have vascular disease or have had a myocardial infarction, but specific improvement in diastolic dysfunction has not been demonstrated [19,20].

Calcium channel blockers and angiotensin receptor blockers are effective antihypertensive agents in elderly patients and may provide symptomatic relief in some patients with diastolic CHF. The beneficial effects of **digoxin** on CHF symptoms and rehospitalization also extend to those with diastolic dysfunction and are an alternative when other therapies are ineffective [16].

Nonpharmacologic Management

Despite numerous advances in the pharmacotherapy of heart failure, management of the disease in older persons is difficult. It is often complicated by multiple comorbid medical conditions, polypharmacy, dietary concerns, and psychosocial and financial issues. These can be addressed through a multidisciplinary approach incorporating physicians and nonphysicians. This includes a nurse coordinator or case manager, dietitian, social worker, and clinical pharmacist. Various models have been studied [21].

SHORT-TERM INTERVENTION. One predischarge and one postdischarge visit is provided by a nurse and/or pharmacist in patients hospitalized with heart failure.

SERIAL CONTACTS. An extended series of contacts with a single health care professional, usually a nurse, is provided.

INTEGRATED APPROACH. The integrated approach involves a specific program incorporating physicians, nurses, dietitians, and social workers that work with a patient over many months.

HEART FAILURE TEAM. Comprehensive management is provided by a specialized heart failure/transplant team, often at an academic medical center.

Of note, improving access to primary care services without a focused intervention is not effective [22].

The goals of multidisciplinary management are patient education; promoting self-management skills; improving medication and dietary compliance; encouraging daily weight measurements and exercise; and providing close follow-up through telephone contacts, home health, and office visits. The nonphysicians on the team can perform many of these tasks. The physician's role is to reduce polypharmacy and drug interactions, simplify medical regimens by switching to once-daily medications when possible, and lead the multidisciplinary team.

The impact of this approach is profound and has been validated in randomized controlled trials in elderly patients and confirmed in a metaanalysis [22,23]. The effect on rehospitalization and quality of life is equivalent in magnitude to that observed in clinical trials of ACE inhibitors, beta blockers, and digoxin [21]. Most of the methods studied are also cost-effective [22]. A mortality advantage has not been demonstrated.

ARRHYTHMIAS

Advanced age is associated with an increased frequency of supraventricular, ventricular, and bradyarrhythmias. However, diagnosis and treatment are often the same in younger and older individuals. There are a few basic principles that apply to elderly patients, as well as a few syndromes that require special consideration. Syncope is discussed elsewhere in this text (see Chap. 8, Dizziness, Syncope, and Orthostatic Hypotension).

The symptoms of an arrhythmia can be nonspecific, such as fatigue, shortness of breath, and impaired cognition, or classic palpitations and syncope. This is important because often the decision to implant a pacemaker depends on the presence of symptoms.

Medications and polypharmacy are particularly common causes of bradyarrhythmias in older persons. Often, beta blockers, calcium channel blockers, and digoxin are the agents involved, but clonidine and ophthalmic beta blockers should also be considered.

Age is not a contraindication to placement of a pacemaker or implantable cardioverter-defibrillator. In fact, most of these devices are placed in patients >65 yrs.

When choosing a drug treatment and the choice between devices, consider the patient's wishes, life expectancy, and expected quality of life. For instance, implantation of an implantable cardioverter-defibrillator to reduce the risk of sudden death might contradict a patient's wish for the dying process. Also, the risk of antiarrhythmic drug toxicity is greater in the elderly and can limit the benefits of treatment.

ATRIAL FIBRILLATION

AF is the most common and clinically important arrhythmia in older persons. The prevalence doubles with each decade after the age of 50 yrs to approximately 10% of octogenarians, with a median age of 75 yrs [24]. In the elderly, it is usually associated with underlying cardiac disease such as HTN, coronary artery disease, valvular disease, and sick sinus syndrome (SSS). Transient or reversible causes include cardiac surgery, alcohol, hyperthyroidism (see Chap. 18, Thyroid Disease in the Geriatric Patient), stimulants such as theophylline, pericarditis, acute myocardial infarction, and electrolyte abnormalities, especially hypokalemia and hypomagnesemia.

History

Older persons with AF present with a range of symptoms, from mild palpitations to acute pulmonary edema or stroke. Many are completely asymptomatic with the diagnosis only being made on a routine ECG or physical exam. Other symptoms include fatigue, dizziness, dyspnea, poor exercise tolerance, syncope, and angina.

Management

Complications: Thromboembolic Stroke
For many patients, the major sequela of AF is the risk of an ischemic stroke. It is five times higher than the general population, at approximately 5%/year [25]. Furthermore, in the Framingham Heart Study, the proportion of strokes attributable to AF increased from 1.5% in patients aged 50–59 yrs to 23.5% after age 80 yrs [26].

Treatment
The goal of therapy is to minimize the hemodynamic consequences of AF and to reduce the risk of stroke. The acute treatment of symptomatic AF with rapid ventricular response is the same in older and younger patients.

RATE CONTROL. Control of the ventricular rate is required to minimize the symptoms of AF. As the rate increases, left ventricular filling declines, which exacerbates the already impaired filling due to the loss of atrial contraction and decreased ventricular compliance. This can be particularly detrimental in older persons in whom as much as 30–40% of left ventricular end-diastolic volume may be attributable to the atrial kick [27]. AF often leads to overt CHF.

Rate control can be achieved with any agent that prolongs conduction through the atrioventricular node. **Beta blockers** and nondihydropyridine calcium channel blockers are commonly used oral medications. **Diltiazem** may be better tolerated than **verapamil** because of a lower incidence of hypotension and constipation. **Digoxin** is a useful option in patients with left ventricular dysfunction but is ineffective in patients with hyperthyroidism, a fever, or other conditions with increased sympathetic tone. **Amiodarone** is very effective, but because of its side effects should be limited as a rate-controlling agent to patients in whom other medications are ineffective or contraindicated.

Dosing of these medications is similar in older and younger patients. It is important to recognize drug interactions that require modifying the dose, especially with digoxin, amiodarone, and warfarin.

RHYTHM CONTROL. The consequences of AF can theoretically be eliminated through electrical or pharmacologic cardioversion to and subsequent maintenance of normal sinus rhythm. Unfortunately, antiarrhythmic agents are only modestly effective at maintaining sinus rhythm and have not been shown to reduce stroke risk or overall mortality. Until data from more trials are available, repetitive attempts at rhythm control should be reserved for patients who have highly symptomatic AF despite attempts at rate control.

ANTICOAGULATION. The benefits of anticoagulation to prevent stroke in patients with chronic AF have been demonstrated in numerous randomized controlled trials and a metaanalysis. Long-term therapy with warfarin or ASA reduces a patient's chance of having a stroke by 68% and 21%, respectively. However, the risk of intracranial bleeding increases with advancing age, and data addressing anticoagulation therapy in patients >75 yrs are limited. There are also no well-validated methods to weigh the benefits of stroke prevention against the risk of bleeding in an individual patient. These principles should be considered when determining the best anticoagulation therapy for a specific patient:

- **Significant contraindications** to warfarin therapy include a recent intracranial hemorrhage, active bleeding, and serious noncompliance. Managing warfarin therapy requires regular follow-up of a patient's INR to ensure correct dosing of the medication. The risk of bleeding in patients >75 yrs dramatically increases with an INR >3.0 [28].
- **Although the chance of intracranial bleeding increases as people age, so does their risk of stroke, and the percentage of those strokes attributable to AF increases. Therefore, the actual number of strokes prevented may increase as people age.**
- An individual's stroke risk can even be determined with a validated instrument such as the CHADS$_2$ index [29]. This tool for understanding pertinent risk factors for stroke may help a physician and his or her patient decide about antithrombotic therapy.
- **Fall risk is often cited as a relative contraindication to warfarin therapy, but there is no evidence to support this decision.** In fact, based on available epidemiologic and trial data, a decision analysis found that an **individual would need to fall almost 300 times per year to outweigh the benefits of warfarin therapy** [30]. Until better information is available, physicians should be cautious of withholding antithrombotic therapy simply because of the risk of falls (see Chap. 7, Falls).
- **If warfarin therapy is not chosen, all patients should at least be treated with ASA.** Low-dose warfarin therapy + ASA is no more effective than ASA alone [31].

SICK SINUS SYNDROME

SSS is a syndrome of sinoatrial dysfunction usually found in elderly patients. The prevalence may be as high as 1 in 600 patients >65 yrs, and it accounts for 50% of pacemaker implantations [32].

Increasing age is associated with a decline in the number of functioning pacemaker cells in the sinus node and degeneration of the conduction system in the atria and through the atrioventricular node. This manifests as a combination of both supraventricular tachyarrhythmias and bradyarrhythmias. This includes AF and flutter, sinus bradycardia, sinus pauses and arrest, sinus exit block, advanced atrioventricular nodal block, and AF with a slow ventricular response. **A common scenario is the tachybrady syndrome in which a tachyarrhythmia such as AF abruptly stops followed by a long sinus pause due to overdrive suppression.** This scenario can be highly symptomatic and predispose to embolic phenomenon.

Symptoms and Evaluation

SSS characteristically presents with nonspecific symptoms of **fatigue, confusion, palpitations, or syncope.** Thus, correlating symptoms with ECG documentation of arrhythmias is important. A single ECG is often insufficient, so a **24-hr Holter monitor or patient-activated event recorder** can be used. Rarely, invasive electrophysiologic testing is necessary to make the diagnosis.

Once SSS is identified, it is necessary to identify any extrinsic causes of sinus node dysfunction and treat them. These include hypothyroidism, hypothermia, electrolyte imbalances, increased intracranial pressure, and drugs that produce sinus node dysfunction. These include beta blockers, calcium channel blockers, digoxin, clonidine, and antiarrhythmic agents such as amiodarone.

Treatment

The goal of treatment is to eliminate the bradyarrhythmias, which cause most of the symptoms in SSS, and reduce the frequency of tachyarrhythmias. However, patients with SSS are particularly susceptible to the bradycardic effects of medications used to treat tachyarrhythmias. Thus, the mainstay of treatment in patients who are highly symptomatic is **cardiac pacing** along with a **beta blocker, calcium channel blocker, digoxin, or other antiarrhythmic agent to suppress tachycardia.** For patients in sinus rhythm, dual-chamber pacing is associated with a better quality of life than single-chamber ventricular pacing [33]. In patients with chronic or paroxysmal AF as part of their SSS, anticoagulation is indicated.

AORTIC STENOSIS

Valvular disease is common in elderly patients. Aside from stenotic lesions of the aortic valve, evaluation and management of other lesions are similar in younger and older patients. AS is the most common valvular disorder requiring surgery in the elderly. It affects 2–3% of patients >65 yrs and increases in prevalence with age [34,35].

Pathophysiology

In most elderly patients, the pathogenesis is an active disease process similar to atherosclerosis that leads to calcification and thickening of the trileaflet aortic valve [36]. **In 25% of patients older than 65 yrs, this manifests as aortic sclerosis in which there is no obstruction to blood flow across the valve** [34,35]. **This is not a benign condition and is associated with a 50% increase in the risk of death from cardiovascular causes and the risk of myocardial infarction** [37]. A significant subset of these patients will slowly progress to clinically significant **AS** requiring valve replacement. Once symptoms develop, 2-yr survival rates are <50% without surgery [36].

Diagnosis

AS in the elderly is often occult. The classic symptoms and physical exam findings of AS include CHF, angina, syncope, decreased carotid upstroke, S4, and a systolic murmur at the base radiating to the carotids. However, **sedentary older persons may**

experience few symptoms until their disease is far advanced or attribute their symptoms to old age or to other illnesses. Similarly, physicians often attribute these nonspecific symptoms to other causes. **It is also difficult to rule out AS based on auscultation alone** [38]. The murmur may be less prominent, secondary to changes in chest wall geometry and a reduced stroke volume. As a result of decreased vascular compliance, carotid upstrokes can be preserved. The critical point is that **whenever unexplained symptoms could be secondary to AS, echocardiography should be pursued.** Cardiac catheterization is indicated in patients with severe AS who are candidates for surgery.

Management

Before the development of symptoms, the same basic management principles apply to younger and older patients with AS. This includes **endocarditis prophylaxis,** avoidance of vigorous physical activity with moderate to severe AS, and avoidance of excessive preload reduction. Careful follow-up with a thorough clinical assessment and echocardiography is necessary every 6–12 mos to monitor for symptoms and disease progression.

Aortic valve replacement (AVR) is the treatment of choice in elderly patients with symptomatic AS. Asymptomatic patients should very rarely be considered for an AVR, as there is no demonstrated benefit [36]. Optimally, surgery should be performed at the onset of symptoms because preop CHF negatively effects late survival after surgery [39]. This can be especially difficult in the elderly because of potentially nonspecific symptoms and should include consultation with a specialist. It is also important to consider the impact of dementia, advanced frailty, and major comorbidities while helping patients and their families decide about surgery.

The outcome of AVR in the symptomatic elderly is excellent compared to the dismal prognosis without surgery, even in octogenarians. Perioperatively, mortality rates range from 4–8% in several series but are higher when AVR is combined with coronary artery bypass graft [40]. The majority of patients experience marked improvement in their symptoms, functional capacity, long-term survival and quality of life comparable to the general population of similar age [39].

KEY POINTS TO REMEMBER

- Heart failure is predominantly a geriatric syndrome that has become a major public health concern in the twenty-first century because of the aging population.
- A distinguishing feature of heart failure in the elderly is the high prevalence of cases that occur in the setting of normal or near-normal left ventricular function.
- As no single clinical feature can reliably distinguish between a systolic or diastolic cause for heart failure, an assessment of left ventricular function is essential.
- Frequent monitoring is an essential part of treating elderly patients with heart failure.
- To date, no large trials of a specific therapy for diastolic dysfunction have been completed. Pharmacologic management is empiric and should be guided by prevailing comorbidities and symptomatic relief.
- A multidisciplinary team approach to treating heart failure, incorporating physicians and nonphysicians, leads to significant improvements in rehospitalization and quality of life.
- AF is the most common and clinically important arrhythmia in older persons.
- Fall risk is often cited as a relative contraindication to warfarin therapy, but there is no evidence to support this decision.
- Sedentary older persons may experience few symptoms of AS until their disease is far advanced or attribute their symptoms to old age or to other illnesses.
- It is also difficult to rule out AS based on auscultation alone. Whenever unexplained symptoms could be secondary to AS, echocardiography should be pursued.
- The outcome of AVR in the elderly is favorable compared to the dismal prognosis without surgery.

SUGGESTED READING

ACC/AHA guidelines for the management of patients with valvular heart disease: a report of the American College of Cardiology/American Heart Association Task Force on Practice Guidelines (Committee on Management of Patients with Valvular Heart Disease). *J Am Coll Cardiol* 1998;32:1486–1588.

Akins CW, Daggett WM, Vlahakes GJ, et al. Cardiac operations in patients 80 years old and older. *Ann Thoracic Surg* 1997;64:606–615.

Cheitlin MD, Gerstenblith G, Hazzard WR, et al. Do existing databases answer clinical questions about geriatric cardiovascular disease and stroke? *Am J Geriatr Cardiol* 2001;10:207–223.

The European Atrial Fibrillation Trial Study Group. Secondary prevention in nonrheumatic atrial fibrillation after transient ischaemic attack or minor stroke. *Lancet* 1993;342:1255–1262.

Gruppo Italiano per lo Studio della Sopravvivenza nell'Infarto Miocardio: GISSI-3: Effects of lisinopril and transdermal glyceral trinitrite singly and together on 6-week mortality and ventricular function after acute myocardial infarction. *Lancet* 1994;343:1115–1122.

Kober L, Torp-Pedersen C, Carlsen JE, et al. A clinical trial of the angiotensin-converting-enzyme inhibitor trandolapril in patients with left ventricular dysfunction after myocardial infarction. Trandolapril Cardiac Evaluation (TRACE) Study Group. *N Engl J Med* 1995;333:1670–1676.

Laupacis A, Boysen G, Connoly S, et al. The efficacy of aspirin in patients with atrial fibrillation: analysis of pooled data from 3 randomized trials. *Arch Intern Med* 1997;157:1237–1240.

Levy D, Larson MG, Vasan RS, et al. The progression from hypertension to congestive heart failure. *JAMA* 1996;275:1557–1562.

Pfeffer MA, Braunwald E, Moye LA, et al. Effect of captopril on mortality and morbidity in patients with left ventricular dysfunction after myocardial infarction. *N Engl J Med* 1992;327:669–677.

The SOLVD Investigators. Effect of enalapril on survival in patients with reduced left ventricular ejection fractions and congestive heart failure. *N Engl J Med* 1991;325:293–302.

Wong WF, Gold S, Fukuyama O, et al. Diastolic dysfunction in elderly patients with congestive heart failure. *Am J Cardiol* 1989;63:1526–1528.

REFERENCES

1. Rich MW. Heart failure in the 21st century: a cardiogeriatric syndrome. *J Gerontol A Biol Sci Med Sci* 2001;56(2):M88–M96.

1a. American Heart Association. *Heart disease and stroke statistics. 2003 update.* Dallas: AHA, 2002.

2. Kannel WB, Belanger AJ. Epidemiology of heart failure. *Am Heart J* 1991;121: 951–957.

3. National Heart, Lung, and Blood Institute. Congestive heart failure in the United States: a new epidemic. Bethesda, MD: U.S. Department of Health and Human Services, 1996. Available at: http://www.nhlbi.nih.gov/health/public/heart/other/chf_abs.htm. Accessed May 2003.

4. Graves EJ, Owings MF. 1995 Summary: National Hospital Discharge Survey. Advance data from vital and health statistics; no. 291. Hyattsville (MD): National Center for Health Statistics, 1997.

5. O'Connell JB, Bristow MR. Economic impact of heart failure in the United States: time for a different approach. *J Heart Lung Transplant* 1994;13:S107–S112.

6. Vasan RS, Larson MG, Benjamin EJ, et al. Congestive heart failure in subjects with normal versus reduced left ventricular ejection fraction: prevalence and mortality in a population based cohort. *J Am Coll Cardiol* 1999;33:1948–1955.

7. Kitzman DW, Gardin JM, Gottdiener JS, et al. Importance of heart failure with preserved systolic function in patients ≥ 65 years of age. *Am J Cardiol* 2001;87:413–419.

8. Rockwood K. Acute confusion in elderly medical patients. *J Am Geriatr Soc* 1989;37:150–154.
9. Gottdiener JS, Arnold AM, Aurigemma GP, et al. Predictors of congestive heart failure in the elderly: the Cardiovascular Health Study. *J Am Coll Cardiol* 2000;35:1628–1637.
10. Garg R, Yusuf S. Overview of randomized trials of angiotensin-converting enzyme inhibitors on mortality and morbidity in patients with heart failure. *JAMA* 1995;273:1450–1456.
11. Flather MD, Yusuf S, Kaber L, et al. Long-term ACE-inhibitor therapy in patients with heart failure or left-ventricular dysfunction: a systematic overview of data from individual patients. *Lancet* 2000;355:1575–1581.
12. Packer M, Bristow MR, Cohn JN, et al. The effect of carvedilol on morbidity and mortality in patients with chronic heart failure. *N Engl J Med* 1996;334:1349–1355.
13. CIBIS-II Investigators and Committees. The cardiac insufficiency bisoprolol study II (CIBIS II): a randomized trial. *Lancet* 1999;353:9–13.
14. Effect of Metoprolol CR/XL in chronic heart failure. Metoprolol CR/XL Randomised Intervention Trial in Congestive Heart Failure (MERIT-HF). *Lancet* 1999;353:2001–2007.
15. Pitt B, Zannad F, Remme WJ, et al. The effect of spironolactone on morbidity and mortality in patients with severe heart failure. Randomized Aldactone Evaluation Study Investigators. *N Engl J Med* 1999;341:709–717.
16. The Digitalis Investigation Group. The effect of digoxin on mortality and morbidity in patients with heart failure. *N Engl J Med* 1997;336:525–533.
17. Ware JA, Snow E, Luchi JM, et al. Effect of digoxin on ejection fraction in elderly patients with congestive heart failure. *J Am Geriatr Soc* 1984;32:631–635.
18. Cohn JN, Archibald DG, Ziesche S, et al. Effect of vasodilator therapy on mortality in chronic congestive heart failure: results of a Veterans Administrative Cooperative Study. *N Engl J Med* 1986;314:1547–1552.
19. Yusuf S, Sleight P, Pogue J, et al. Effects of an angiotensin-converting-enzyme inhibitor, ramipril, on cardiovascular events in high-risk patients. The Heart Outcomes Prevention Evaluation Study Investigators. *N Engl J Med* 2000;342:145–153.
20. Aronow WS. Management of older persons after myocardial infarction. *J Am Geriatr Soc* 1998;46(11):1459–1468.
21. Kerzner R, Rich MW. Does multidisciplinary management of chronic heart failure improve clinical outcomes? *J Clin Outcomes Manag* 2001;8(2):41–49.
22. McAlister FA, Lawson FME, Teo KK, et al. A systematic review of randomized control trials of disease management programs in heart failure. *Am J Med* 2001;110:378–384.
23. Rich MW, Beckman V, Wittenberg C, et al. A multidisciplinary intervention to prevent the readmission of elderly patients with heart failure. *N Engl J Med* 1995;333:1190–1195.
24. Kannel WB, Wolk PA, Benjamin EJ, et al. Prevalence, incidence, prognosis and predisposing conditions for atrial fibrillation: population-based estimates. *Am J Cardiol* 1998;82:2N–9N.
25. Atrial Fibrillation Investigators. Atrial fibrillation: risk factors for embolization and efficacy of antithrombotic therapy. Analysis of pooled data from five randomized controlled trials. *Arch Intern Med* 1994;154:1449–1457.
26. Wolf PA, Abbott RD, Kannel WB. Atrial fibrillation as an independent risk factor for stroke: The Framingham study. *Stroke* 1991;22:983–988.
27. Aronow WS. Management of older persons with atrial fibrillation. *J Am Geriatr Soc* 1999;47:740–748.
28. The Stroke Prevention in Atrial Fibrillation Investigators. Bleeding during antithrombotic therapy in patients with atrial fibrillation. *Arch Intern Med* 1996;156:409–416.
29. Gage BF, Waterman AD, Shannon W, et al. Validation of clinical classification schemes for predicting stroke: results from the National Registry of Atrial Fibrillation. *JAMA* 2001;285:2864–2870.
30. Man-Son-Hing M, Nichol G, Lau A, et al. Choosing antithrombotic therapy for

elderly patients with atrial fibrillation who are at a risk for falls. *Arch Intern Med* 1999;159:677–685.

31. Stroke Prevention in Atrial Fibrillation Investigators. Adjusted-dose warfarin versus low-intensity, fixed dose warfarin plus aspirin for high-risk patients with atrial fibrillation: Stroke Prevention in Atrial Fibrillation III randomised clinical trial. *Lancet* 1996;348:633–638.

32. Mangrum JM, DiMarco JP. The evaluation and management of bradycardia. *N Engl J Med* 2000;342:703–709.

33. Lamas GA, Orav EJ, Stambler BS, et al. Quality of life and clinical outcomes in elderly patients treated with ventricular pacing as compared with dual-chamber pacing. Pacemaker Selection in the Elderly Investigators. *N Engl J Med* 1998;338:1097–1104.

34. Stewart BF, Sisovick D, Lind BK, et al. Clinical factors associated with calcific aortic valve disease: Cardiovascular Health Study. *J Am Coll Cardiol* 1997;29:630–634.

35. Lindroos M, Kupari M, Heikkila J, et al. Prevalence of aortic valve abnormalities in the elderly: an echocardiographic study of a random population sample. *J Am Coll Cardiol* 1993;21:1220–1225.

36. Otto CM. Aortic stenosis—listen to the patient, look at the valve. *N Engl J Med* 2000;343:652–654.

37. Otto CM, Lind BK, Kitzman DW, et al. Association of aortic-valve sclerosis with cardiovascular mortality and morbidity in the elderly. *N Engl J Med* 1999;341:142–147.

38. Munt B, Legget ME, Kraft CD, et al. Physical examination in valvular aortic stenosis: correlation with stenosis severity and prediction of clinical outcome. *Am Heart J* 1999;137:298–306.

39. Kvidal P, Bergstrom R, Horte LG, et al. Observed and relative survival after aortic valve replacement. *J Am Coll Cardiol* 2000;35:747–756.

40. Tseng EE, Lee CA, Cameron DE, et al. Aortic valve replacement in the elderly. *Ann Surg* 1997;225:793–804.

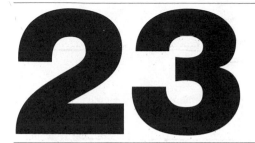

23

**Urologic Symptoms
and Urinary Tract
Infection in
the Elderly**

Sam B. Bhayani

UROLOGIC SYMPTOMS

Urologic symptoms are subdivided into **lower and upper urinary tract symptoms.** Lower urinary tract symptoms are further subdivided into irritative and obstructive symptoms.

Lower Urinary Tract Symptoms

Lower urinary tract symptoms refer to a spectrum of voiding complaints referable to the bladder, urethra, and prostate. The normal adult voids six times a day, has a bladder capacity of 300–400 mL, and is continent between voids. Although urologic disease predominates as a cause of lower urinary tract symptoms, gynecologic, GI, and neurologic etiologies should also be considered. Diabetes mellitus should be excluded as a contributing factor.

→ **Irritative symptoms include frequency, dysuria, urgency, and nocturia.** Causes of irritative voiding include UTI, hyperreflexic neurogenic voiding dysfunction, excessive fluid intake, polyuria, bladder tumor, and bladder calculi. Benign prostatic hyperplasia in men and cystocele in women may produce irritative symptoms or obstructive symptoms.

⇒ **Obstructive symptoms include hesitancy, dribbling, weakened urinary stream, intermittency of urinary stream (stopping and starting), and straining.** Potential causes are benign prostatic hyperplasia, urethral stricture, atonic bladder, obstructing tumor, and cystocele. Obstructive symptoms are usually quantified and followed with the American Urological Association symptom score (see Appendix H).

Incontinence is the unintentional leakage of urine (see Chap. 24, Urinary Incontinence).

*nepheolithiasis → stones. in kidney a canal
myelonephritis → infection of kidney*

Upper Urinary Tract Symptoms

Upper urinary tract symptoms are not specific to the urinary tract. Upper urinary tract symptoms include flank pain, costovertebral angle pain, back pain, nausea, and abdominal pain. Urologic causes include nephrolithiasis, upper tract tumor, ureteral obstruction, and pyelonephritis. Investigation relies on imaging tailored to the history, symptoms, and patient condition. CT scan, renal U/S, and intravenous pyelography are the most useful imaging studies to investigate a urologic cause of these symptoms.

cystitis → bladder infection

URINARY TRACT INFECTION IN THE ELDERLY

Presentation

Risk Factors
Predisposing factors include BPH with resultant urinary stasis, comorbid diseases such as diabetes mellitus, indwelling urinary catheters or external collection devices, immobility, diminished immune response, and neurogenic voiding dysfunction.

History
Symptoms are varied. Acute cystitis can produce incontinence, dysuria, frequency, hematuria, urinary retention, and suprapubic pain. These symptoms are often non-

specific, as many elderly patients have lower urinary tract symptoms related to chronic incontinence, benign prostatic hyperplasia, diabetes mellitus, or neurogenic voiding dysfunction. Fever may be present. Pyelonephritis is associated with fever, flank pain, nausea, emesis, and mental status changes. Elderly patients may present with delirium and no urinary symptoms.

Evaluation and Lab Studies
Male patients and neurologically impaired patients should electively undergo a postvoid residual urine measurement to rule out urinary retention as a correctable etiology. Symptomatic patients should have a UA and culture, blood count, and basic metabolic profile. Close monitoring of serum glucose is necessary in diabetic patients.

Management

Asymptomatic Bacteruria
Asymptomatic bacteruria with pyuria is often present in **ambulatory, institutionalized, and catheterized populations.** Many prospective randomized trials have shown no increase in morbidity or mortality with observation. The presence of pyuria should not influence treatment, as >90% of patients have significant pyuria. Asymptomatic bacteruria should only be temporarily treated if subjects undergo invasive genitourinary procedures.

Symptomatic Urinary Tract Infection
Acute cystitis is generally treated for 7 days in the geriatric population. *Escherichia coli* is the most common organism. Other organisms include *Proteus, Klebsiella, Pseudomonas, Enterococcus,* and other gram-positive organisms. **A pretreatment urine culture is recommended,** because organisms are more varied than in younger populations. Treatment can be with 7 days of trimethoprim-sulfamethoxazole (TMP-SMX) (Bactrim) or a fluoroquinolone.

    Acute pyelonephritis should initially be treated with hospitalization and parenteral therapy. Ampicillin (Principen, Totacillin) (1 g IV q6h) and gentamicin (Garamycin) (5 mg/kg IV qd) are preferred. Quinolones can be substituted, and PO forms have the same bioavailability as IV administration. Outpatient therapy with fluoroquinolones should be considered in healthy patients with no systemic systems.

Recurrent Urinary Tract Infection
Patients with recurrent UTI with urease splitting organisms such as ***Pseudomonas, Klebsiella, and Proteus*** should undergo abdominal x-ray, renal U/S, or CT to rule out struvite urolithiasis.

Epididymo-Orchitis
Epididymo-orchitis may be associated with UTI. *E. coli* is the most common organism in the geriatric population. Treatment consists of 2–4 wks of TMP-SMX or fluoroquinolone. If fever or leukocytosis persists, consider evaluation for a scrotal or prostatic abscess.

KEY POINTS TO REMEMBER

- Risk factors for UTI in the elderly include benign prostatic hyperplasia, diabetes, indwelling urinary catheters or external collection devices, immobility, impaired immunity, and neurogenic voiding dysfunction.
- Delirium may be the presentation of an otherwise asymptomatic UTI in the elderly.
- Postvoid residuals should be performed in older men who develop a UTI.
- Acute cystitis is usually caused by *E. coli* and should be treated with 7 days of antibiotics in the elderly.
- A pretreatment urine culture is advised in the elderly patient with a UTI.

REFERENCE AND SUGGESTED READING

Barnett BJ, Stephen DS. Urinary tract infection: an overview. *Am J Med Sci* 1997; 314:245–249.

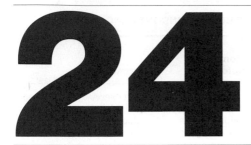

Urinary Incontinence

Sam B. Bhayani

INTRODUCTION

Incontinence is the involuntary leakage of urine. The prevalence increases with age. **Patients are frequently embarrassed about their symptoms and do not volunteer their symptoms without specific questioning.** Some causes of incontinence are transient or medication related. More commonly, incontinence (Table 24-1) is associated with increased intraabdominal pressure (stress urinary incontinence), involuntary bladder contraction (urge urinary incontinence), full bladder (overflow incontinence), urinary fistulae, or neurologic compromise. Patients may exhibit a mixture of types of incontinence. **All patients should undergo UA, post-void residual urine evaluation, and neurologic exam.**

PRESENTATION

History

The first step is to identify the problem, as many patients do not volunteer a history of incontinence. **It should be determined whether the incontinence is new or chronic** (various etiologies of transient incontinence are listed in Table 24-2). Chronic incontinence should be categorized as stress, urge, or overflow incontinence. These types are discussed in detail below. The rest of the history should focus on associated symptoms and diagnoses (especially previous surgeries and deliveries, diabetes mellitus, cognitive dysfunction, and immobility). Specifics about frequency, volume, and timing can be ascertained with a **voiding record. Important medications to inquire about include diuretics, anticholinergic medications, narcotics, alpha blockers, beta blockers, alpha agonists, and calcium channel blockers.** History should also focus on risk factors for skin breakdown (see Chap. 10, Pressure Sores).

Physical Exam

Physical exam should focus on the genitourinary tract and rectum: bladder distension, vaginitis, benign prostatic hyperplasia (BPH), cystocele, rectocele, and fecal impaction should be excluded. **Neurologic exam** should be performed to evaluate cognitive dysfunction as well as sacral reflexes (sphincter tone and anal wink reflex) and perineal sensation. **A post-void residual is a routine part of the evaluation and should be <50 mL.**

Lab Studies

Standard lab evaluation includes electrolytes, calcium, glucose, BUN, Cr, and UA. Urodynamics are not routinely indicated.

TRANSIENT URINARY INCONTINENCE

Transient incontinence occurs in up to one-third of the geriatric population. **Causes can be remembered with the mnemonic DIAPPERS** (Table 24-2).

TABLE 24-1. CLINICAL SUBTYPES OF URINARY INCONTINENCE

Type	Predominate gender affected	Predominate symptoms	Treatment
Stress incontinence	Female	Worse with increased intraabdominal pressure (coughing, laughing, etc.)	Kegel exercises, estrogens, ephedrine, tricyclic antidepressants (imipramine), surgery
Urge incontinence	Both	Urgency	Timed voiding, fluid restriction, anticholinergics if cognitively intact treatment of BPH
Overflow incontinence	Male	Obstructive symptoms, prostatism	Catheterization (intermittent or indwelling), treatment of BPH/obstruction
Functional incontinence	Both	Immobility, cognitive impairment	Behavioral interventions, protective undergarments or pads, environmental modification

BPH, benign prostatic hyperplasia.

STRESS URINARY INCONTINENCE

Stress urinary incontinence occurs when **increased intraabdominal pressure overcomes a weakened urethra or damaged urethral sphincter.** Leakage occurs in the absence of a bladder contraction.

Stress Urinary Incontinence in Women

Etiologies include vaginal delivery, prior gynecologic surgery, deconditioned pelvic musculature, or decreased urethral resistance secondary to diminished estrogen.

History and physical exam reveal leakage with coughing, sneezing, laughing, and exercise. The leakage may be demonstrated by exam with cough or strain when the patient is standing. Hypermobility of the urethra may be noted on pelvic exam.

TABLE 24-2. DIAPPERS MNEMONIC FOR CAUSES OF TRANSIENT URINARY INCONTINENCE

Delirium: incontinence resolves as mental status improves.

Infection: urinary infection can irritate the bladder, causing leakage.

Atrophic vaginitis or urethritis: treated with estrogen replacement.

Pharmaceuticals: many medications can affect voiding pattern, including psychotropic medications, diuretics, anticholinergics, alpha-adrenergic agonists or antagonists, narcotics, calcium channel blockers, and vincristine.

Psychological problems: incontinence is associated with severe depression.

Excess urine output.

Restricted mobility affects ability to reach restroom facilities.

Stool impaction.

Conservative therapy includes fluid restriction, timed voiding q2–3h to keep the bladder empty, and Kegel exercises to strengthen the pelvic floor.

Medical therapy includes conjugated estrogen (0.625 mg PO qd) or topical estrogen (1 g 3 ×/wk) should be considered to encourage urethral perfusion, coaptation, and promote vaginal muscle tone (see Chap. 13, Sex Hormone Therapy in the Elderly Woman). Beneficial effects may start 6 wks after therapy institution. Results are highly variable. Ephedrine (25–50 mg PO tid) and pseudoephedrine (30–60 mg q8h) are alpha sympathomimetic agents that act on urethral smooth muscle to increase outlet resistance. Imipramine (Tofranil) (50–150 mg PO qhs) is a tricyclic antidepressant (TCA) that can increase urethral smooth muscle tone and relax the bladder detrusor muscle. These medications are often ineffective in severe cases of stress urinary incontinence and should be used with caution in the geriatric population.

Surgical referral is indicated if conservative measures fail. Urologists and urogynecologists can perform urethral sling and support procedures to correct urethral hypermobility or intrinsic sphincter deficiency. Long-term success rates are 60–90%, and a short hospitalization is often required.

Stress Urinary Incontinence in Men

Stress urinary incontinence is **rare** in the male patient. The urethra is well supported by the prostate and corpora, and, therefore, leakage with increased intraabdominal pressure is rare. The most common etiology is postprostatectomy, secondary to a compromised internal urethral sphincter. Conservative therapy includes fluid restriction, timed voiding q2–3h, and pelvic floor exercises to strengthen musculature. Medical therapy with ephedrine, pseudoephedrine, and imipramine may also be used (see Stress Urinary Incontinence in Women for doses). In refractory or severe cases, surgical therapy has been successful. Patients can undergo a temporary periurethral collagen injection or undergo implantation of an artificial urinary sphincter.

URGE URINARY INCONTINENCE

Urge urinary incontinence occurs when the bladder involuntarily contracts. Leakage occurs when this unsuppressed contraction overcomes sphincter pressure.

Urge Urinary Incontinence in Women

Etiologies include bladder irritation secondary to infection, radiation, chemotherapy, fecal impaction, and tumor. Neurologic compromise may also cause involuntary bladder contraction. Many cases are idiopathic.

History reveals leakage after an uninitiated urge to urinate that cannot be suppressed. Physical exam should include pelvic and rectal exam. Urge and stress incontinence may coexist.

Conservative therapy includes timed voiding, fluid and diuretic restriction, and oral estrogen (0.625 mg PO qd) or topical estrogen (1 g 3 ×/wk) (see Chap. 13, Sex Hormone Therapy in the Elderly Woman).

Pharmacologic therapy includes anticholinergic agents that suppress bladder contraction. Oxybutynin (Ditropan) (5 mg PO q8h) may be used. **Anticholinergic side effects such as dry mouth, constipation, dry eyes, cognitive dysfunction, and somnolence may be observed.** Newer agents such as oxybutynin XL (5–10 mg PO qd), tolterodine (Detrol) (1–2 mg PO q12h), and tolterodine LA (Detrol LA) (4 mg PO qd) reportedly have fewer side effects but still produce some anticholinergic effects (including cognitive dysfunction) and are more expensive.

Surgical therapy is possible. Urologists may perform bladder augmentation or sacral nerve stimulation to counter the unstable bladder.

Urge Urinary Incontinence in Men

Etiologies include neurologic illness; bladder irritation from infection, calculus, or tumor; or bladder dysfunction from severe BPH.

History reveals leakage after an unsuppressible urge to urinate. Exam should evaluate the prostate and neurologic system. Urinary infection should be ruled out. Conservative measures such as fluid restriction and timed voiding can limit incontinent episodes.

Pharmacologic therapy includes the use of anticholinergic agents such as those outlined in Urge Urinary Incontinence in Women. Note that urge incontinence can be secondary to irritation from BPH. Anticholinergic agents should be used with extreme caution in elderly male patients, as they may precipitate urinary retention in men with BPH, in addition to other undesirable effects. Post-void residual urine should be regularly checked in all elderly male patients on anticholinergics. Generally, BPH should be treated before urge incontinence, as it may be the cause of irritative voiding symptoms (see Chap. 25, Benign Prostatic Hyperplasia, Erectile Dysfunction, and Prostate Cancer).

OVERFLOW URINARY INCONTINENCE

Overflow urinary incontinence is assessed by measuring the post-void residual urine (normal, <50 mL). Patients retain urine and are unable to empty their bladders.

Overflow Urinary Incontinence in Men

Etiologies include anatomic obstruction from benign prostatic hypertrophy or urethral stricture. An acontractile bladder may be secondary to diabetes mellitus or neurologic illness. Medications with anticholinergic side effects may also cause urinary retention. Examples include antihistamines, TCAs, alpha agonists, narcotics, and antispasmodics.

History may reveal a pattern of obstructive voiding symptoms, such as straining, dribbling, weak urinary stream, and urinary frequency. Patients usually leak a small amount of urine at frequent intervals. A history of urethral manipulation and sexually transmitted diseases should be elicited. Exam may reveal an enlarged prostate. Neurologic exam should be performed. An American Urological Association symptom score is usually assigned and used to follow the patient's symptoms (see Appendix H).

Treatment is based on emptying the bladder. Acutely, an indwelling catheter or intermittent catheterization may be instituted. Further therapy is targeted at the etiology of retention. If the Cr is elevated, a renal imaging should be performed to rule out hydronephrosis from chronic outlet obstruction.

BPH is treated with medications or surgery (see Chap. 25, Benign Prostatic Hyperplasia, Prostate Cancer, and Erectile Dysfunction).

Retention secondary to neurologic illness or diabetes mellitus is best treated with clean intermittent catheterization. Alternatively, an indwelling catheter or suprapubic tube can be placed.

Overflow Urinary Incontinence in Women

Overflow urinary incontinence in women is uncommon and usually represents an underlying peripheral neuropathy. Diabetes mellitus is the most common cause. Patients should be placed on clean intermittent catheterization. In selected cases, an indwelling Foley catheter or suprapubic tube may be a reasonable option.

FUNCTIONAL URINARY INCONTINENCE

Functional urinary incontinence occurs in frail elderly patients and may coexist with other types of incontinence. Patients may be unwilling (depression, hostility) or unable (dementia, immobility) to maintain continence. Treatment should focus on identifying and treating reversible contributing factors as well as other types of incontinence. Most of the other interventions are implemented by the caregivers, such as scheduled voiding on a regular basis, reinforcement of the patient's current voiding habits, frequent prompting to urinate, and removal of environmental barriers. **Risk of skin breakdown** should be assessed with appropriate preventative action taken (see Chap. 10, Pressure Sores). Use of protective undergarments or padding may be useful, and special circumstances may warrant indwelling urinary catheterization.

KEY POINTS TO REMEMBER

- Many patients do not offer a history of urinary incontinence without specific questioning.
- The history should focus on the onset of symptoms, medications, comorbid illnesses, and bladder habits.
- Causes of transient incontinence should be evaluated (DIAPPERS mnemonic).
- Physical exam includes a careful genitourinary, rectal, and neurologic evaluation.
- Stress urinary incontinence usually occurs in women and is associated with leaking of urine with increased intraabdominal pressure (cough, sneeze, etc.).
- Overflow incontinence typically occurs in men with obstructive symptoms and prostatic disorders.
- Urge incontinence is due to involuntary bladder contractions, which may respond to anticholinergic agents.
- Functional incontinence frequently occurs in frail elderly patients as a consequence of cognitive impairment, immobility, or other inability to toilet effectively.
- Management of incontinence should include conservative measures such as scheduled voiding, fluid restriction, and removal of offending medications.

REFERENCES AND SUGGESTED READINGS

Chutka SD, Fleming KC, Evans MP, et al. Urinary incontinence in the elderly population. *Mayo Clin Proc* 1996;71:93–101

Ouslander JG, Johnson TM. Incontinence. In: Hazzard WR, ed. *Principles of geriatric medicine and gerontology.* New York: McGraw-Hill, 1998.

25

Benign Prostatic Hyperplasia, Erectile Dysfunction, and Prostate Cancer

Sam B. Bhayani

BENIGN PROSTATIC HYPERPLASIA

Introduction

Benign prostatic hyperplasia (BPH) is a condition in which the bladder outlet is obstructed by an enlarged prostate. 25–50% of men >65 yrs are affected [1].

History and Physical Exam

Patients with BPH may present with a variety of obstructive and irritative voiding symptoms. Hesitancy, weak stream, straining, urgency, frequency, nocturia, and urinary retention may be present. **To quantify BPH, a symptom index** has been developed by the American Urological Association [2] (see Appendix H). **Physical exam may reveal a suprapubic distended bladder or an enlarged prostate.** Neurologic exam should be performed to rule out voiding dysfunction secondary to neurologic illness.

Management

Lab Studies

Studies should include a UA and culture, as the symptoms of BPH may coexist with infection. Prostate-specific antigen (PSA) may be checked to evaluate for prostate cancer, but the value can be falsely elevated with urinary retention, recent urinary catheterization, or digital rectal exam. Uroflowmetry or urodynamics testing may be considered by urologists to distinguish BPH from urgency or neurogenic voiding dysfunction.

Treatment

Therapy is tailored to the severity of the symptoms. **Conservative measures are indicated in all patients with BPH.** Fluid restriction and elimination of diuretics and caffeinated products before travel or sleep can reduce nocturia and frequency.

Pharmacologic therapy falls in two major classes of medications: alpha blockers and 5-alpha reductase inhibitors.

Prostatic smooth muscle responds to alpha-adrenergic stimulus. Alpha-adrenergic blockade has been shown to increase urinary flow rates and decrease symptom scores by up to 50% [3]. **Terazosin (Hytrin)** is started at 1 mg PO qhs and titrated up to 5–10 mg PO qhs over 2–3 wks. Side effects are dose related and include **orthostatic hypotension, dizziness,** nasal congestion, peripheral edema, and **syncope. Doxazosin (Cardura)** is started at 1 mg PO qhs and increased to 8 mg PO over 2–3 wks. Side effects are similar to terazosin. **Tamsulosin (Flomax) (0.4 mg PO qhs) is a highly selective alpha blocker with fewer cardiovascular side effects, so dose titration is not necessary.**

Finasteride (Proscar) (5 mg PO qd) is a 5-alpha reductase inhibitor that reduces intraprostatic dihydrotestosterone levels, theoretically limiting prostatic growth. Treatment is necessary for 6 mos before effects are seen. Its efficacy in treating BPH is controversial. The Proscar Long-Term Efficacy and Safety Study [4] (PLESS trial) was a double-blinded, randomized, placebo-controlled trial of 3040 patients treated with finasteride or placebo. It showed a statistically significant reduction in risk of >50% for acute urinary retention (10% placebo, 5% with finasteride) and need for

BPH surgery (7% with placebo, 3% with finasteride) with the use of finasteride over 4 yrs. Critics of the study contend that >90% of patients do not benefit from finasteride and are treated unnecessarily at a significant cost. **Recent trials show that finasteride is most effective in patients with markedly enlarged prostates and has little use in patients with mild enlargement** [5]. The VA cooperative study #359 [6] compared finasteride, terazosin, and placebo in a 1229-patient randomized double-blind trial. Finasteride was found to be similar to placebo in the treatment of BPH, whereas terazosin and the combination of terazosin and finasteride offered similar reductions in the American Urological Association symptom score and increases in peak urinary flow rates. **Side effects of finasteride include loss of libido and erectile dysfunction (ED).** Finasteride causes a reduction in PSA. **For prostate cancer screening, the patient's actual PSA is doubled and therefore is considered elevated when >2.**
Surgical therapy is the preferred treatment of severe or refractory BPH:

- **Conservative surgical therapy** is available in the outpatient setting. Transurethral microwave therapy and thermotherapy have been shown to moderately improve BPH symptoms with minimal side effects.
- **Transurethral resection of the prostate is the standard surgical therapy.** Patients' satisfaction rates are >90%, and most patients can stop BPH medications after surgery. **Side effects include retrograde ejaculation in most patients, impotence (5%), and incontinence (1%).**
- Open prostatectomy is reserved for extremely large glands in which transurethral surgery is not feasible.

ERECTILE DYSFUNCTION

Introduction
ED is defined as the inability to maintain penile rigidity sufficient for sexual relations. It is a very common disorder in the geriatric population [7].

Etiology
Erection requires integration of psychogenic, neurologic, vascular, and hormonal processes. Dysfunction in any of these processes may induce ED. **Often in the elderly patient, ED is multifactorial.** Medications may also induce ED. Many cases are idiopathic:

- **Psychogenic** causes include depression, stress, and anxiety.
- **Neurologic** causes include cerebrovascular accident, peripheral neuropathy, parkinsonian disorders, and postprostatectomy ED.
- **Vascular** causes of ED include atherosclerosis or cavernosal venous leak.
- **Hormonal** causes include hyperprolactinemia and androgen deficiency (see Chap. 12, Androgen Deficiency in Older Men).
- **Medications causing ED** include antihypertensives, antiandrogens, anticholinergics, and psychotropics.

Presentation
History
A complete medical and sexual history should be taken. Medications and tobacco use should be documented. Evidence of neuropathy, atherosclerosis, depression, or HTN should be investigated. An assessment of the patient's libido should be made.
    ED symptoms can be assessed with the SHIM (Sexual Health Inventory for Men; Appendix I).

Physical Exam
Physical exam can help to reveal the etiology of ED. **Hormonal ED may be associated with gynecomastia and loss of axillary or suprapubic hair. Bitemporal hemianopsia may indicate a pituitary mass.** The abdomen should be examined for evidence of

hepatic or vascular disease. **Genitourinary exam should evaluate for penile plaques, testicle size, and phallic sensation.** Diminished peripheral and femoral pulses may indicate vascular disease. Neurologic evaluation should include assessment of perineal and perianal sensation and peripheral motor and sensory nerve assessment.

Management

Lab Evaluation
All patients should have routine blood count, electrolyte assessment, and glucose level checked to evaluate for major systemic illnesses. Routine hormonal testing for hypogonadism in men with ED is controversial. Hypogonadism is a rare cause of ED, and hormonal testing is expensive. However, libido may be an inaccurate clinical assessment of testosterone levels. An early-morning testosterone level may be checked; if abnormal, further evaluation with prolactin, free testosterone, luteinizing hormone, FSH, and testosterone-binding globulin may be indicated (see Chap. 12, Androgen Deficiency in Older Men).

Diagnostic Studies
Generally, diagnostic studies are not indicated, as they frequently **do not change overall management.** Nocturnal penile tumescence studies can separate psychogenic impotence from organic causes. If psychogenic impotence is suspected, patients will continue to have nocturnal erections that can be monitored in a sleep lab. Penile brachial index studies may indicate arteriogenic impotence if the value is <0.75. Penile duplex U/S can also assess flow and venous leak. Other studies include cavernosometry and cavernosography to assess vascular ED. Neurologic testing may include biothesiometry and electromyelography studies.

Treatment
A variety of treatments are available for patients with ED. Because of its ease of administration and efficacy, sildenafil (Viagra; 25–100 mg PO) is generally the first-line therapy before extensive evaluation. Other options are available, and urologic consultation should be considered in many cases.

   Sildenafil is a selective inhibitor of type 5 cyclic guanosine monophosphate phosphodiesterase. It functions by enhancing nitric oxide–mediated smooth muscle relaxation in the glans and corpora, with resultant increase in flow and rigidity of the phallus. In the absence of stimulation, its effects are not significant. Sildenafil is available in 25-mg, 50-mg, and 100-mg doses. **Time to peak plasma concentration is a median of 60 mins,** and efficacy is optimal on an empty stomach. In placebo-controlled trials involving >3000 patients with mixed causes of ED, improvement in erections was noted in up to 82% of patients [8].

- **Dosage usually starts at 50 mg PO 1 hr before intercourse.** If no effect, 100 mg may be tried at a different time. In worldwide flexible dose studies, 60% of patients ultimately selected the 100-mg dose [9]. The 25-mg dose should be considered in patients with significant hepatic dysfunction.
- **Side effects include headache, flushing, dyspepsia, nasal congestion, and abnormal blue-tinged or hazy vision.**
- **Sildenafil is absolutely contraindicated in patients using nitrates regularly or intermittently.** The FDA has cautioned against use of sildenafil in patients who have generally been excluded from clinical trials, such as patients with **history of myocardial infarction, stroke, hypotension, and retinitis pigmentosa.**

   Intraurethral alprostadil (PGE1) comes with an applicator to introduce a small pellet of alprostadil as an intraurethral suppository. The medicine is absorbed and induces corporeal smooth muscle relaxation and rapid arterial inflow. Dosages are 125 µg, 250 µg, 500 µg, and 1000 µg. Efficacy is highly variable, with improved erections in 30–75% of patients. Side effects include local penile pain, urethral bleeding, and dizziness. There are few contraindications because it is not systemically absorbed and can be used in patients with cardiac disease.

Intracavernosal injection therapy is the most effective therapy for ED. Therapy is usually instituted under the supervision of a urologist. The patient is instructed on self-injection of intracavernosal prostaglandin, phentolamine, or papaverine. Up to 87% of patients obtain erections satisfactory for intercourse [10], with highest responses noted for those with vasculogenic impotence. Complications include priapism, penile pain, and fibrosis.

Vacuum erection devices are a nonpharmacologic option. Patients are instructed on the fit and use of the device by their physician, urologist, and manufacturer's representative. Success rates range from 30–70%, but discontinuation is common secondary to pain, lack of spontaneity, or unnatural feelings. A relative contraindication is anticoagulant therapy.

Testosterone therapy may be indicated for patients with low testosterone levels. Oral preparations are associated with hepatotoxicity, and **transdermal therapy is preferred.** Testosterone therapy should be used with caution in the geriatric population, as androgens may speed prostatic growth and potentiate prostatic carcinoma (see Chap. 12, Androgen Deficiency in Older Men).

Surgical penile prosthesis implantation is a safe and effective solution in many patients. Satisfaction rates are >80%.

PROSTATE-SPECIFIC ANTIGEN SCREENING AND PROSTATE CANCER

Prostate-Specific Antigen Screening

PSA is a nonspecific marker for prostate cancer. Elevation is possible with BPH, prostate manipulation, prostatitis, and prostate cancer.

Although nonspecific, it is the **best marker for the detection of prostate cancer.** Before PSA screening, only 30% of men with prostate cancer had organ-confined disease [11]. With screening and early detection, 60–80% of men have organ-confined disease and are potentially curable [12,13].

The most widely accepted indication for prostate biopsy is a PSA ≥4. Some urologists use PSA velocity, PSA density, lower PSA cutoffs, or age-specific PSA ranges to decide on prostatic biopsy.

The American Cancer Society recommends digital rectal exam and PSA screening for all patients at age 50 yrs who have a >10-yr life expectancy [14]. African American patients and patients with a family history of prostate cancer should undergo screening at age 45. **Most urologists stop screening at age 70–75 yrs, as prostate cancer is conservatively treated in most of these patients.**

Free PSA can improve the sensitivity of PSA screening. Patients with prostate cancer have a lower amount of unbound PSA. A free PSA percentage of ≤25% improves the sensitivity of PSA screening [15]. This is clinically useful in patients reluctant to undergo biopsy, patients with multiple benign biopsies and an elevated PSA, and patients near the 4.0 cutoff.

Prostate Cancer

Prostate cancer is the **most common malignancy in men.** Treatment options should be **individualized** based on patient health, comorbidity, and patient preference.

Treatment of Clinically Localized Prostate Cancer

Radical prostatectomy is reserved for patients <70 yrs who are in excellent health and have life expectancy of >15 yrs. The surgery can be performed from retropubic, perineal, or laparoscopic approaches. Side effects include incontinence in 5–20% and impotence in 20–70%. Long-term data on survival appears excellent, with 70% progression-free survival at 10 yrs [16].

Radiotherapy may be performed with external beam radiotherapy or brachytherapy. Both are efficacious for treatment of clinically localized disease. Controversy exists as to whether radiation therapy is as efficacious as radical prostatectomy, with conflicting studies. Advantages are primarily the noninvasive nature of the treatment.

Side effects include impotence in 20–40%, irritative voiding complaints in 10–20%, and radiation proctitis in 2%. Brachytherapy may have fewer side effects than external beam radiotherapy.

Hormonal therapy may be used for clinically localized prostate cancer. Hormonal therapy seeks to lower serum testosterone levels to suppress prostatic cancer growth. Hormonal therapy is palliative, and there is controversy as to whether hormonal therapy at an early stage offers survival advantage over hormonal therapy used at a later stage. Nevertheless, some patients desire therapy. Hormonal therapy is discussed in greater detail below.

Watchful waiting is a reasonable option in patients with <10-yr life expectancy and low-grade tumors. PSA should be followed q6mos. If PSA rises consistently or symptoms develop, therapy can be instituted.

Treatment of Locally Advanced Prostate Cancer and Metastatic Disease
External beam radiation therapy has been used for locally advanced prostate cancer when there is no evidence of metastasis. 10-yr survival rates are 10–30%.

Hormonal therapy is the mainstay of advanced prostate cancer. Prostate cancer is androgen dependent, and hormonal therapy seeks to lower testosterone to castrate levels to slow cancer growth.

- **Orchiectomy is the most cost effective method of androgen ablation,** but some patients prefer medical castration.
- **Luteinizing hormone-releasing hormone (LHRH) agonists (leuprolide, goserelin)** temporarily stimulate luteinizing hormone and testosterone production, then suppress luteinizing hormone release within 2 wks and, subsequently, lower testosterone levels to castrate levels. They are offered as injections or implants lasting 3 mos, 4 mos, or 1 yr.
  - **The flare response** is an acute exacerbation of clinical symptoms (obstructive voiding, bony pain) from the initial rise in testosterone. This flare can be blocked by a peripherally acting antiandrogen such as flutamide (Eulexin) (250 mg PO tid), bicalutamide (Casodex) (50 mg PO qd), or nilutamide (Nilandron) (100 mg PO qd).
  - **Intermittent therapy can be offered to patients with LHRH agonists.** Therapy is instituted until PSA becomes undetectable and then stopped for many months until PSA rises. Preliminary studies show equivalent survival to constant androgen blockade, but patients spend nearly 50% of time off therapy.
- **Side effects of androgen deprivation therapy include hot flashes, loss of libido, osteoporosis, and other symptoms of androgen deficiency** (see Chap. 12, Androgen Deficiency in Older Men). **Calcium and vitamin D supplementation along with bisphosphonates should be considered in patients undergoing hormonal therapy.**
- Blockade of adrenal androgens has been used to complement testosterone blockade. Adrenal androgens are converted to testosterone in the prostate. Nonsteroidal antiandrogens such as flutamide, bicalutamide, and nilutamide competitively bind to the testosterone receptor. Randomized trials have been conflicting, but currently there is no evidence that blockade of adrenal androgens lengthens survival. Antiandrogens, however, can lower rising PSA in patients with advanced hormone-resistant prostate cancer.

Complications of Advanced Prostate Cancer
Bony pain limits quality of life in prostate cancer patients. Specific metastasis can be palliated with a 2- to 3-wk course of external beam radiation with improvement in 75% of patients. Strontium-89 injection can also improve pain in 50% of cases. Consultation with radiation oncologists should be considered.

Spinal cord compression is an emergency and should be suspected in any patient with advanced prostate cancer and neurologic compromise. Evaluation consists of spinal MRI or CT. Treatment should involve immediate androgen ablation if the patient has not been previously treated. LHRH agonists should be avoided secondary to their associated androgen flare response. Orchiectomy or ketoconazole (Nizoral) (400 mg PO tid) prevents testosterone production. Glucocorticoid replacement is necessary during ketoconazole administration. Steroid therapy and emergent spinal radiation can decompress the spinal cord. Surgical decompression may be necessary in severe cases.

KEY POINTS TO REMEMBER

- The incidence of ED, BPH, and prostate cancer increases with age.
- BPH presents with obstructive and irritative symptoms and is diagnosed clinically.
- The American Urological Association symptom score can be useful for diagnosing BPH, assessing the severity of symptoms, and monitoring the effects of therapy.
- Medical treatment for BPH includes alpha blockers (i.e., tamsulosin) and 5-alpha reductase inhibitors (finasteride). Finasteride is only beneficial in patients with large prostates after at least 6 mos of treatment.
- Surgical therapy results in symptomatic improvement for most patients with BPH with some risk of complications, including retrograde ejaculation, ED, and incontinence.
- ED has many potential etiologies and is usually multifactorial in the elderly.
- Most men with ED can be effectively treated.
- Although prostate cancer is common in the elderly, most men with cancer do not die from it.
- The decision to screen for prostate cancer must be individualized. Most clinicians stop screening for prostate cancer after the age of 75 yrs and in those with life expectancies of <10 yrs.
- Clinically localized prostate cancer can be surgically cured, treated with hormonal therapy, or followed with a "watchful waiting" approach. More advanced disease can be treated with radiation and/or hormonal therapy.

SUGGESTED READING

DeBusk R, et al. Management of sexual dysfunction in patients with cardiovascular disease: recommendations of the Princeton Consensus Panel. *Am J Cardiol* 2000;86:175–181.

Dull P, Reagan RW, Bahnson RR. Managing benign prostatic hyperplasia. *Am Fam Physician* 2002;66:77–84, 87–88.

Harris R, Lohr KN. Screening for prostate cancer: an update of the evidence for the U.S. Preventative Task Force. *Ann Intern Med* 2002;137:917–929.

Lue TF. Erectile dysfunction. *N Engl J Med* 2000;342:1802–1813.

U.S. Preventative Task Force. Screening for prostate cancer: recommendation and rationale. *Ann Intern Med* 2002;137:915–916.

REFERENCES

1. Chute CG, et al. The prevalance of prostatism: a population-based survey of urinary symptoms. *J Urol* 1993;150:85–89.
2. Barry MJ, et al. The American Urological Association symptom index for benign prostatic hyperplasia. *J Urol* 1992;148:1549–1557.
3. McConnell JD, et al. Benign prostatic hyperplasia: diagnosis and treatment. Clinical practice guideline, number 8. AHCPR Publication No. 94-0852. Rockville, MD: Agency for Health Care Policy and Research, Public Health Service, U.S. Department of Health and Human Services, 1994.
4. McConnell JD, et al. The effect of finasteride on the risk of acute urinary retention and the need for surgical treatment in men with benign prostatic hyperplasia. *N Engl J Med* 1998;338:557–563.
5. Boyle P, et al. Prostate volume predicts outcome of treatment of BPH with finasteride: meta-analysis of randomized controlled trials. *Urology* 1996;48:398–405.
6. Lepor H, et al. The efficacy of terazosin, finasteride, or both in benign prostatic hyperplasia. *N Engl J Med* 1996;335:533–539.
7. Feldman HA, et al. Impotence and its medical and psychosocial correlates: results of the Massachussetts male aging study. *J Urol* 1994;151:54–61.

8. Fink HA, et al. Sildenafil for male erectile dysfunction. A systemic review and meta-analysis. *Arch Intern Med* 2002;162:1349–1360.
9. Padma-Nathan H, Giuliano F. Oral drug therapy for erectile dysfunction. *Urol Clin North Am* 2001;28:321–334.
10. European Alprostadil Study Group. The long-term safety of alprostadil (Prostaglandin-E1) in patients with erectile dysfunction. *Br J Urol* 1998;82:538–543.
11. Thompson IM, Ernst JJ, Gangai MP, et al. Adenocarcinoma of the prostate: results of routine urological screening. *J Urol* 1984;172:690–692.
12. Smith DS, Catalona WJ. The nature of prostate cancer detected through prostate specific antigen based screening. *J Urol* 1994;152:1732–1736.
13. Catalona WJ, Smith DS, Ratliff TL, et al. Detection of organ-confined prostate cancer is increased through prostate-specific antigen-based screening. *JAMA* 1993;270(8):948–954.
14. Smith RA, Cokkinides V, von Eschenbach AC, et al. American Cancer Society guidelines for the early detection of cancer. *CA Cancer J Clin* 2002;52(1):8–22.
15. Catalona WJ, Partin AW, Slawin KM, et al. Use of the percentage of free prostate-specific antigen to enhance differentiation of prostate cancer from benign prostatic disease: a prospective multicenter clinical trial. *JAMA* 1998;279(19):1542–1547.
16. Krongrad A, Lai H, Lai S. Survival after radical prostatectomy. *JAMA* 1997; 278(1):44–46.

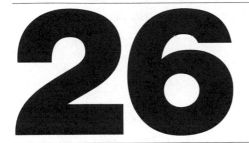

Parkinson's Disease and Related Disorders

Kyle C. Moylan

INTRODUCTION

The diagnosis and management of Parkinson's disease (PD) in the elderly are challenging. Both the disease and its treatment can have dramatic effects on cognitive and physical functioning. >1 million Americans are affected by PD, making it the second most common neurodegenerative disorder [Alzheimer's disease (AD)] being the most common). **The classic features of parkinsonism are tremor, rigidity, and bradykinesia.** Parkinsonism is a syndrome with multiple possible causes and must be distinguished from PD.

Parkinsonism is especially common in the geriatric population, as age is the most consistent risk factor. It affects 15% of the population at age 65 yrs and approximately 50% of the population at age 85 yrs [1]. Although multiple disorders with parkinsonian features have now been described, **idiopathic PD is ten times as common as atypical parkinsonian disorders**. Parkinsonism can be caused by idiopathic PD, drugs, head trauma, Wilson's disease, cerebrovascular disease, hydrocephalus, multisystem atrophy (MSA), dementia with Lewy bodies (DLB), cortical basal ganglionic degeneration (CDGD), progressive supranuclear palsy (PSP) and advanced AD. The clinical features are the only means of distinguishing between PD and the atypical parkinsonian disorders. There is considerable overlap among these disorders in clinical practice, and many patients do not clearly fit into one disorder. When possible, determining the specific diagnosis is important, because the prognosis and response to treatment vary substantially. **Underdiagnosis of parkinsonism is common,** which is unfortunate, because effective treatment can improve quality of life. In addition, mortality is 2–5 times higher in PD patients than their peers [1].

PATHOPHYSIOLOGY

PD is a neurodegenerative disorder of uncertain etiology. Most cases are sporadic, although 10% of cases have a familial component. Pathologically, it is characterized by progressive neuronal death leading to formation of Lewy bodies (composed of degenerating neuronal processes and containing alpha-synuclein). Destruction of the dopaminergic cells in the substantia nigra is central to the motor dysfunction, although cholinergic cells in the nucleus basalis of Meynert and other cells in the brain stem, hypothalamus, cortex, and autonomic nuclei are also affected. Some loss of dopaminergic neurons and dopamine synthesis occurs with usual aging. **The size of the substantia nigra pars compacta decreases with age, and this decrease is associated with poor performance on motor tasks** [2]. This cell loss is accelerated in PD and more selectively affects the putamen. Concomitant AD pathology is not unusual in the elderly with PD.

PRESENTATION

Clinical Features of Parkinson's Disease

The presence of two of the three classic parkinsonian signs is highly suggestive of PD. Onset is usually insidious after the age of 50. Other features that suggest a diagnosis of PD include a sustained and significant response to an adequate trial of levodopa,

TABLE 26-1. HOEHN AND YAHR STAGING OF PARKINSON'S DISEASE

Stage 1

Signs and symptoms on one side only

Symptoms mild

Symptoms inconvenient but not disabling

Usually presents with tremor of one limb

Stage 2

Friends have noticed changes in posture, locomotion, and facial expression

Symptoms are bilateral

Minimal disability

Posture and gait affected

Stage 3

Significant slowing of body movements

Early impairment of equilibrium on walking or standing

Generalized dysfunction that is moderately severe

Stage 4

Severe symptoms

Can still walk to a limited extent but usually requires assistance

Rigidity and bradykinesia

No longer able to live alone

Tremor may be less than earlier stages

Stage 5

Cachectic stage

Invalidism complete

Cannot stand or walk

Requires constant nursing care

From Hoehn MM, Yahr MD. Parkinsonism: onset, progression, and mortality. *Neurology* 1967;17:427–442, with permission.

postural instability, and a slowly progressive course. **A patient probably does not have PD if the symptoms evolve rapidly or if the patient responds poorly to levodopa.** The clinical stages have been outlined by Hoehn and Yahr [3] (Table 26-1). **Motor symptoms usually start in one limb, and then spread to the other limb on the affected side.** Bilateral involvement can then occur, but symptoms usually remain asymmetric until the late stages.

Older patients tend to have earlier impairment of posture and gait than their younger counterparts, whereas younger patients have more dyskinesias and motor fluctuations [4].

History

The history should first ascertain **when the symptoms first began** and **on which side of the body.** Patients typically present with motor symptoms such as tremor, although these may be predated by nonspecific symptoms such as fatigue, malaise, depression, and personality changes. Inquire about current and past exposure to antipsychotics and related antiemetics (see Drug-Induced Parkinsonism).

Rest tremor affects 75% of patients with PD at presentation [5] and occurs less often in atypical disorders. The parkinsonian tremor is characterized as **pinrolling** and usually starts in one arm. It increases with anxiety (like all tremors) and sympathomimetics but abates during motor actions or sleep.

Bradykinesia, akinesia, and rigidity may manifest as symptoms of motor slowing or loss of facial expression. **Specific tasks to inquire about include any difficulty rising from a chair, opening jars, using buttons, turning in bed, or change in handwriting (micrographia)** [6]. Some slowing occurs with normal aging; for example, one-fourth of older adult pedestrians are unable to traverse a crosswalk in the time allotted by traffic signals [7].

The voice may be softer or muffled. Dysarthria can occur late in the course.

Shuffling gait, postural instability, and falls are common and occur earlier in the elderly. Patients may have difficulty starting or stopping their gait, known as **start hesitation** and **propulsion,** respectively. Motor freezing may be noted when going through doorways.

Nonmotor symptoms are often overlooked but are common. Early onset of nonmotor symptoms may suggest an atypical parkinsonian disorder (see below).

Neuropsychiatric Abnormalities

Neuropsychiatric abnormalities are **particularly common** in the elderly.

Cognitive dysfunction (see Parkinson's Disease and Cognitive Dysfunction) can range from mild impairment to severe dementia. Unlike AD, memory is relatively preserved. The history may reveal difficulty performing complex tasks and problem solving (executive dysfunction) as well as cognitive slowing (bradyphrenia).

Depression may affect up to 60% of patients with PD at some time during the course of the disease [8]. Some symptoms, such as lack of energy, psychomotor slowing, and sleep disturbances, may be due to PD or depression. Consider using a structured interview or a screening tool, such as the Geriatric Depression Scale (see Chap. 5, Depression in the Older Adult, and Appendix C), for evaluating these symptoms at baseline and over time. Both anxiety and depression can occur during "off" periods and respond best to adjustment of antiparkinsonian medications to reduce off time.

Hallucinations are usually related to antiparkinsonian medications and can affect up to 30% of treated patients [9]. Patients usually report seeing people or animals, particularly at night or in shadows. Usually patients retain insight that these are indeed hallucinations and antipsychotic treatment may not be needed. Early psychosis not related to treatment is usually not PD but is common with diffuse Lewy body disease (DLBD).

Sleep disturbances are common.

Autonomic Dysfunction

Autonomic dysfunction usually occurs later in the course of PD and is prominent early in MSA.

Particularly concerning is orthostatic hypotension, which can lead to immobility and falls. It can be disease or treatment related.

Dysphagia can occur in later stages and may be an important cause of weight loss.

Impotence is typically a late feature of PD but may occur early in other disorders.

Constipation is almost universal. Nocturia, urinary frequency, and incontinence occur frequently and are caused by detrusor hyperactivity.

Sensory Disturbances

Sensory disturbances can occur and include anosmia, numbness, aching, and paresthesias.

Physical Exam

The physical exam should focus on the typical motor findings [6]. The examiner should be alert to the pattern of these features, such as any asymmetry or involvement of the axial musculature. The timing of the most recent dose of antiparkinsonian medication should be recorded in relation to the exam. Rating tools such as the Unified Parkinson's

Disease Rating Scale subscale III (see Appendix O) can be used to standardize the physical exam and quantify the severity of the findings. This is particularly useful for following the patient over time and assessing the response to treatment.

Tremor must be distinguished from other etiologies, particularly essential tremor (ET), which is also common in the elderly. **Tremor at rest is usually parkinsonian.** The tremor of ET tends to be more symmetric and pronounced during posture or action (writing, holding a cup or utensil). The tremor can usually be elicited by having the patient rest his or her hands in the lap, particularly if distracted by having them recite serial 7s. When tremor affects the head, PD patients usually have a flexion-extension tremor (nodding yes) whereas patients with ET usually shake the head left and right (shaking no). The tremor of PD is slow, with a frequency of 3–5 Hz, but all tremors tend to be slower in the elderly, and this may not be a useful distinguishing feature.

Rigidity is increased muscle tone present throughout the entire range of passive motion. **Cogwheeling** may or may not be present. Each limb and the neck should be tested independently. When rigidity is mild, it can be accentuated by asking the patient to move the contralateral side. Rigidity must be distinguished from spasticity (flexor muscles in the arms and extensor muscles in the legs preferentially affected), contractures (actual shortening of muscle fibers), and paratonia (involuntary resistance to passive movement, common in patients with dementia).

Bradykinesia and akinesia are prominent features, defined as slowness or paucity of movement. The examiner can test finger tapping, hand movements, and heel tapping. Overall, bradykinesia and akinesia can be observed throughout the history taking and physical exam, including **masked facies.** As mentioned, some symmetric slowing of movement occurs with usual aging.

Have the patient try to stand from a seated position with his or her arms folded across the chest. Patients with parkinsonism may arise slowly, need more than one attempt, or be unable to complete the task. Proximal muscle weakness and arthritis can cause similar difficulties.

The characteristic gait disorder is a stooped posture with short, shuffling steps; a narrow base; and reduced arm swing. Start hesitation, festination, (progressively smaller and more rapid steps as the body leans forward), **propulsion** (difficulty stopping once the gait is initiated), and **freezing** (especially during turns or passing through doorways) may be observed. Turns may be accomplished through a series of small, short steps or by moving the body as a single unit (*en bloc*). Gait impairment is common in the elderly and can occur from a variety of causes. Short steps and flexed posture can be seen with senile gait disorder, usually with a wide base. The flexed posture can be mimicked by osteoporosis, kyphosis, and other spinal abnormalities.

Postural instability can be assessed using the **pull test** but is unnecessary if spontaneous postural instability is observed. The patient stands in front of the examiner, who explains how the test is performed. The examiner should pull the patient backward with a single forceful thrust (the examiner must be prepared to catch the patient). An abnormal postural response is noted if the patient cannot maintain their balance with one or two steps backward.

Cognitive assessment should be performed at baseline in the elderly and periodically thereafter, particularly if there is a history suggesting cognitive decline (see Appendix A).

BP should be measured supine, sitting, and standing.

Eye movements are examined for limitations in eye movements, abnormal saccades, and impaired accommodation.

PARKINSON'S DISEASE AND COGNITIVE DYSFUNCTION

Some degree of cognitive dysfunction is detectable in almost all patients with PD when extensive neuropsychometric testing is performed, even in untreated patients. The disturbances may be subclinical or result in disabling dementia. These disturbances are not necessarily progressive and may not correlate with the development of dementia. **The presence of dementia is associated with more rapid progression of illness, poorer motor response to dopaminergic agents, increased**

confusion and hallucinations due to antiparkinsonian medications, higher mortality, and increased caregiver burden [8]. Dementia more commonly leads to institutionalization than do the motor features of PD.

Dementia occurs six times more often in patients with PD than their peers [10] and
is diagnosed when cognitive function impairs daily functioning. The prevalence of
dementia in PD is estimated to be 30–40%. Patients at the greatest risk of developing
dementia are older patients and those with more severe motor symptoms, gait abnormality, and postural instability. PD dementia has been characterized as a subcortical
dementia. Typical abnormalities include **impaired executive function, bradyphrenia,
depression, impaired visuospatial processing, and mild memory impairment.** Language abilities are usually preserved, although speech production can be affected.
Cognitive screens may show normal results or mild impairment.

**AD occurs commonly in older patients with PD, with half of the patients meeting
neuropathologic criteria for AD at autopsy.** It is unclear whether this is merely
related to the high prevalence of both disorders in the elderly or whether there are
shared underlying mechanisms (possibly involving alpha synuclein). Concomitant AD
should be suspected in cases with more memory impairment along with other cortical
deficits such as aphasia or apraxia (see Chap. 3, Dementia).

**Demented patients with PD represent a heterogeneous group that may present
with a wide range of cognitive deficits.** Many patients do not clearly fit into one cate-
gory, and many overlap syndromes are described (Lewy body variant of AD, DLBD, etc.).

DIFFUSE LEWY BODY DISEASE OR DEMENTIA WITH LEWY BODIES

DLBD is now recognized as the second most common cause of neurodegenerative
dementia. **The central features of DLB include cognitive decline, early visual hallucinations (within a year of cognitive dysfunction), and parkinsonism** [11]. The age
of onset (60–85 yrs) is somewhat later than PD.

It is unclear whether DLBD represents a distinct pathologic entity or part of a spectrum of PD with dementia. The distinction between DLBD and PD is based largely on
the timing of the cognitive abnormalities in relation to the parkinsonism (occurring
within 1 yr).

Visual hallucinations occur in approximately one-half of patients but may be
underreported. **The hallucinations may be spontaneous or precipitated by treatment of the parkinsonian symptoms.** Olfactory and auditory hallucinations occur
less frequently, as do systematic delusions.

The **parkinsonism** may be more symmetric, and tremor is less common than with
PD. The response to levodopa is generally suboptimal [12]. **Treatment of hallucinations with neuroleptics may worsen parkinsonism.** Parkinsonism was not a requirement to make the diagnosis in the last consensus guidelines [11].

The **cognitive deficits** are similar to PD (see Parkinson's Disease and Cognitive
Dysfunction) and are progressive.

There is more fluctuation in cognitive performance than with AD. Sometimes,
these fluctuations may be severe and result in transient depression of alertness or
even frank syncope.

Repeated falls are common early in the course (usually a later finding in PD).

DRUG-INDUCED PARKINSONISM

Any drug that inhibits dopamine metabolism or action can induce parkinsonism.
Most drug-induced parkinsonism (DIP) is caused by neuroleptic agents due to D_2 receptor blockade. High-potency neuroleptics such as haloperidol (Haldol) and fluphenazine
(Prolixin) are the most likely to induce DIP, but it can also occur with atypical antipsychotics such as risperidone (Risperdal) and related antiemetics [prochlorperazine (Com-
pazine), promethazine (Phenergan), metoclopramide (Reglan)]. **Elderly women are at
higher risk for developing DIP. Clinically, it tends to be symmetric but may be indistinguishable from idiopathic PD.** 90% of cases develop **within 3 mos of starting therapy** [13]. DIP usually resolves within a few weeks of discontinuing the offending agent.

Prolonged symptoms after drug discontinuation (up to 1 yr) should raise concern for an underlying parkinsonian disorder.

MULTIPLE SYSTEM ATROPHY

MSA represents a conglomerate of olivopontocerebellar atrophy, striatonigral degeneration, and Shy-Drager syndrome.

Patients tend to be younger (median age of onset is 55 yrs) with faster progression (50% are wheelchair bound within 5 yrs).

Parkinsonism is present at onset in approximately one-half of patients. The parkinsonism is usually asymmetric with absent or mild tremor.

Almost all patients develop autonomic dysfunction, which is the presenting symptom in 40% of patients. Impotence is the most common feature in men, and urinary incontinence is most common feature in women.

Orthostatic hypotension is common and frequently requires treatment with fludrocortisone or midodrine. Hypotension can be severe enough to result in complete immobility. Other features include stridor, dysarthria, dysphagia, contractures, peripheral neuropathy, dystonia, and sleep disorders. **Severe dementia is unusual.**

Patients may initially respond to levodopa, but the response is usually not sustained.

PROGRESSIVE SUPRANUCLEAR PALSY

PSP may be misdiagnosed as PD early in the course.

Patients usually present between the ages of 50 and 70 yrs. **Most patients present with parkinsonism,** usually symmetric rigidity and bradykinesia. Axial and proximal rigidity become prominent with impaired gait and postural instability. **Frequent falls occur early on.**

Eye movements may be normal or minimally abnormal initially. Several years into the disease, **oculomotor dysfunction becomes prominent with impaired downward gaze.**

Severe dementia is rare, although frontal lobe dysfunction, emotional incontinence, and depression have been described.

Dysarthria can be severe and may lead to complete anarthria in some patients. **Dysphagia** can also be severe and may necessitate a feeding tube.

Levodopa is effective for up to one-half of patients, particularly for treating the rigidity and bradykinesia. The response is typically modest or brief and may require >1000 mg of levodopa daily. Physical and speech therapy can be beneficial.

CORTICAL-BASAL GANGLIONIC DEGENERATION

CBGD typically presets with asymmetric clumsiness and dystonic posturing of the arm and hand.

Common parkinsonian signs include unilateral limb rigidity, bradykinesia, and postural instability. When tremor is present, it is usually more pronounced with action or posture and subsides with rest.

Unilateral limb dystonia can progress to the "alien limb phenomena" or "useless limb" in 50% of patients. Other features include apraxia, limb levitation, and cortical sensory deficits.

Oculomotor dysfunction, dysarthria, and dysphagia are occasional features.

Dementia can be prominent and is occasionally the presenting feature, with clinical and pathologic overlap with frontotemporal dementia. Aphasia is common.

Parkinsonism is usually refractory to treatment. Botulinum toxin and stretching can be used for associated dystonia.

MANAGEMENT

Lab Studies and Neuroimaging

The diagnosis of parkinsonian disorders is clinical. No lab studies or imaging tests are useful to make the diagnosis, although neuroimaging can be is indicated if there is suspected cerebrovascular disease or hydrocephalus.

Treatment

Optimal management of PD in the elderly takes into account the effects on all domains of functioning, including mobility, cognition, mood, and independence. **Support groups** are available (American Parkinson's Disease Association). Local chapters may offer informational classes, exercise opportunities, and counseling services. **Regular physical activity and stretching** should be encouraged. Patients with gait impairment may benefit from physical therapy for gait training and use of adaptive devices. Other measures to prevent falls should be undertaken (see Chap. 7, Falls). **Depression should be recognized and treated.** No specific agents are preferred in PD other than the general guidelines given for treating depression in the elderly in Chap. 5, Depression in the Older Adult. Antidepressants have rarely been reported to worsen parkinsonism, but this should not be the sole reason for withholding potentially beneficial treatment. Antidepressants with liquid formulations may be preferred for patients with swallowing problems.

Hallucinations may not require any treatment. If hallucinations are severe, upsetting or disturbing behavior, medication adjustment may be necessary. **When possible, gradually reduce the antiparkinsonian medications** [first anticholinergics, then dopa agonists, amantadine, catechol methyltransferase (COMT) inhibitors, and, lastly, levodopa]. Rapid discontinuation of any of these agents can precipitate severe parkinsonism or neuroleptic malignant syndrome. If medication adjustment is not successful, antipsychotic treatment should be used with caution. Antipsychotics have the potential to worsen parkinsonism for weeks or months, even with a single dose. Clozapine (Clozaril) is the safest antipsychotic with regard to its extrapyramidal effects, but rare agranulocytosis limits its widespread use. Alternatively, **quetiapine** (Seroquel) is a newer atypical antipsychotic that predominately works through nondopaminergic pathways and appears to have a low incidence of extrapyramidal effects. The starting dose is 25 mg once or twice daily.

Orthostatic hypotension can complicate PD or MSA and can also be related to medications. Management is no different than for other causes of orthostatic hypotension (see Chap. 8, Dizziness, Syncope, and Orthostatic Hypotension).

Dementia can be treated with cholinesterase inhibitors (see Chap. 3, Dementia), although data are limited. Decreased cholinergic neurotransmission and degeneration of the nucleus basalis occur in PD and DLBD patients with dementia. There is a potential for worsening parkinsonism (particularly tremor), but patients with some DLBD have shown superior responses of cognitive function compared to patients with AD [14].

Motor features of PD usually require treatment. *There is debate about what drug should be used for the initial treatment of PD and when treatment should be initiated* [15]. Concerns exist regarding the potential neurotoxicity of levodopa and its propensity for motor fluctuations. Nevertheless, levodopa remains the most efficacious and safe treatment for the elderly. **Rapid dose decreases or abrupt cessation of antiparkinsonian medications can precipitate severe parkinsonism and neuroleptic malignant syndrome.**

Levodopa is a precursor of dopamine that effectively crosses the blood–brain barrier. It is decarboxylated in the brain and peripheral tissues to form dopamine. Levodopa is administered with carbidopa (Sinemet) to prevent this conversion in peripheral tissues and the associated nausea.

- **Dosing:** several dosage forms are available with varying proportions of levodopa and carbidopa. The daily dose of levodopa is typically 300–2000 mg PO, divided in three to four doses.
- A usual **starting dose** for an elderly patient is carbidopa/levodopa (Sinemet) 25/100, one-half tablet PO three times daily. However, up to 200 mg of carbidopa may be required daily to prevent nausea, and extra carbidopa may be needed (Lodosyn) when using small doses of Sinemet.
- The amount of levodopa should be titrated up by increasing one of the daily doses by a one-half tablet every week until side effects develop or the desired effect occurs.
- **Common side effects** include nausea, anorexia, orthostatic hypotension, somnolence, hallucinations, confusion, sleep disturbances, and vivid dreams.

- Administering carbidopa/levodopa with food may improve the nausea but may decrease drug bioavailability. If nausea persists, supplemental carbidopa (Lodosyn) may be necessary if the patient is receiving <200 mg PO qd. Antiemetics such as prochlorperazine, promethazine, and metoclopramide should be avoided because of their extrapyramidal effects. Ondansetron (Zofran), granisetron (Kytril), or domperidone (Motilium) can be used safely.

- Giving the last dose several hours before bedtime (with dinner) usually improves the vivid dreams or nightmares, but some patients have nocturnal symptoms that require nighttime doses of levodopa.

- **Carbidopa/levodopa (Sinemet CR)** is a longer-acting formulation that is usually not needed for initial therapy. Doses available are 25/100 (unscored) and 50/200 (scored). The bioavailability is 70% of the regular Sinemet, requiring a 30% dose increase if the patient is switched to Sinemet CR. Absorption is more erratic, onset of action is slower, and the drug still requires dosing twice to four times daily.

- **Motor fluctuations:** initially, levodopa is associated with a sustained response (long-duration effect) with no variability in motor performance from dose to dose. Within 5 yrs of treatment, many patients develop motor fluctuations. These may include wearing off (benefit of treatment wears off before the next dose) and the on-off effect (dramatic and sometimes unpredictable fluctuations in mobility and parkinsonism). This is typically managed by increasing the frequency of levodopa administration as often as needed to offset this response.

- **Dyskinesias** (chorea or dystonia) also develop within several years of treatment but tend to be more problematic in younger patients. Dystonia in the lower one-half of the body (i.e., leg cramps) is usually an off-period phenomenon that responds to levodopa. In contrast, upper body dystonia (i.e., cervical dystonia) is usually levodopa induced and may necessitate a dose reduction. Chorea most commonly occurs at the peak effect of levodopa, when the patient's parkinsonism is best treated. Diphasic dyskinesias (chorea) occur as the dose of levodopa first takes effect, subside at peak levels, and return again as the drug wears off. The patient may not complain of chorea even when it is severe, but it is usually noticed by family members.

Dopamine agonists are less effective than levodopa for treating parkinsonism but have a longer duration of action and may carry less risk of dyskinesias [16]. Older dopamine agonists include bromocriptine (Parlodel), pergolide (Permax), and cabergoline (Dostinex). Newer dopamine agonists such as pramipexole (Mirapex) and ropinirole (Requip) have largely replaced the older agents. Dopamine agonists can be used as **initial monotherapy** or as **adjunctive treatment with levodopa.** However, side effects limit their use in the elderly even in low doses, primarily because of delirium, hallucinations, and excessive somnolence.

- **Dosing:** the starting dose should be low and titrated to the desired effect or limiting side effects in weekly intervals: pramipexole, starting dose of 0.125 mg PO, two to three times daily, increasing by 0.125 mg/dose every week up to 4.5 mg daily; and ropinirole, starting dose of 0.25 mg PO two to three times daily, increasing by 0.25 mg/dose every week up to 24 mg daily.

- **Side effects** are pronounced in the elderly and include delirium, hallucinations, cognitive impairment, excessive somnolence, weight gain, postural hypotension, and syncope. When used in combination with levodopa, they may exacerbate side effects due to dopaminergic activity, including dyskinesias.

Amantadine (Symmetrel) probably exhibits its effects through interactions with N-methyl-D-aspartate receptors, although the exact mechanism of action is unknown. It is not nearly as effective as levodopa for the treatment of parkinsonism and is rarely used as monotherapy. It is most useful as adjunctive therapy with levodopa in the elderly, in whom it may improve parkinsonism while reducing motor fluctuations and dyskinesias.

- **Dosing** starts at 100 mg PO twice daily and can be increased slowly up to 400 mg PO daily. The desired effect may take up to 2 wks.

- Elimination is primarily through renal excretion, and **dose adjustment is necessary with renal impairment.**
- **Side effects** include delirium, nausea, insomnia, edema, and livido reticularis.

Selegiline (Eldepryl) is an irreversible MAO-B inhibitor and inhibits the breakdown of dopamine. It has modest effects on parkinsonism and is sometimes used as initial monotherapy to delay the use of levodopa for several months. Selegiline also potentiates the effects of levodopa. It does not slow the progression of disease.

- **Dosing:** the usual dose is 5 mg PO given at breakfast and lunch.
- **Side effects** include insomnia (selegiline is metabolized to amphetamine and methamphetamine), which is why it is given early in the day. Other side effects include dyskinesias, psychosis, and delirium.
- **Interactions:** MAO-B inhibitors do not interact with tyramine-containing foods but rarely can precipitate hypertensive crisis and the serotonin syndrome if given with TCAs, SSRIs, or meperidine.

COMT inhibitors also prevent the breakdown of dopamine. Available agents are tolcapone (Tasmar) and entacapone (Comtan). These drugs are usually used for patients with problematic wearing-off and are given to extend the duration of action of levodopa and reduce off time. They have the potential to worsen dyskinesias and other levodopa side effects (levodopa dose reduction may be necessary). Hepatotoxicity has been reported with tolcapone and liver function test monitoring is recommended. Other side effects of COMT inhibitors include nausea, diarrhea, and discolored urine.

Anticholinergic drugs have limited efficacy in the treatment of parkinsonism and should generally be avoided in the elderly because of the cognitive effects. Examples include trihexyphenidyl (Artane) and benztropine (Cogentin).

Surgical treatment (deep brain stimulator, pallidotomy, thalamotomy) can be beneficial for selected patients, although advanced age precludes surgical therapy at most centers. Optimal candidates have few comorbidities and intact cognitive capabilities. Referral to a surgical center can be considered for patients with severe motor fluctuations and dyskinesias, inability to tolerate effective doses of antiparkinsonian medications, and refractory tremor. Although patients can usually reduce the dose of antiparkinsonian medications, continued medical treatment is typically necessary.

KEY POINTS TO REMEMBER

- Parkinsonism is common in the elderly and has many potential etiologies.
- Idiopathic PD is the most common cause of parkinsonism.
- PD in the elderly is associated with more gait impairment, postural instability, and dementia as compared with younger PD patients.
- Depression affects many patients with PD and should be treated.
- DLB is characterized by early cognitive impairment, visual hallucinations, parkinsonism, falls, syncope, and a fluctuating but gradually progressive course.
- DIP may be indistinguishable from idiopathic PD.
- The safest and most efficacious treatment for motor symptoms in the elderly is levodopa.
- Most patients with PD respond to an adequate trial of levodopa, but common side effects should be anticipated and treated.
- Psychosis and hallucinations can be safely treated without worsening parkinsonism using novel antipsychotic drugs, notably quetiapine and clozapine.

SUGGESTED READING

Ahlskog JE. Parkinson's disease: medical and surgical treatment. *Neurol Clin* 2001;19:579–605.
Lang AE, Lozano AM. Medical progress: Parkinson's disease—first of two parts. *N Engl J Med* 1998;339:1043–1052.

Lang AE, Lozano AM. Medical progress: Parkinson's disease—second of two parts. *N Engl J Med* 1998;339:1130–1143.

Mahant PR, Stacy MA. Movement disorders and normal aging. *Neurol Clin* 2001;19:553–563.

McKeith IG, Burn D. Spectrum of Parkinson's disease, Parkinson's dementia, and Lewy body dementia. *Neurol Clin* 2001;18:865–883.

Siderowf A. Parkinson's disease: clinical features, epidemiology, and genetics. *Neurol Clin* 2001;19:565–578.

REFERENCES

1. Bennett DA, Beckett LA, Murray AM, et al. Prevalence of parkinsonian signs and associated mortality in a community population of older people. *N Engl J Med* 1996;334:71–76.
2. Pujol J, Junque C, Vendrell P, et al. Reduction of the substantia nigra width and motor decline in aging and Parkinson's disease. *Arch Neurol* 1992;49:1199–1122.
3. Hoehn MM, Yahr MD. Parkinsonism: onset, progression, and mortality. *Neurology* 1967;17:427–442.
4. Gibb WR, Lees AJ. A comparison of clinical and pathological features of young- and old-onset Parkinson's disease. *Neurology* 1988;38:1402–1406.
5. Hughes AJ, Daniel SE, Blankson S, et al. A clinicopathologic study of 100 cases of Parkinson's disease. *Arch Neurol* 1993;50:140–148.
6. Rao G, Fisch L, Srinivasan S, et al. The rational clinical examination: Does this patient have Parkinson's disease? *JAMA* 2003;289:347–353.
7. Howie RE, Rubenstein LZ. Are older persons allowed enough time to cross intersections safely? *J Am Geriatr Soc* 1994;24:207–213.
8. Glosser G. Neurobehavioral aspects of movement disorders. *Neurol Clin* 2001;19:535–551.
9. Sanchez-Ramos JR, Ortoll R, Paulson GW. Visual hallucinations associated with Parkinson's disease. *Arch Neurol* 1996;53:1265–1268.
10. Mayeux R, Chen J, Mirabello E, et al. An estimate of the incidence of dementia in idiopathic Parkinson's disease. *Neurology* 1990;40:1513–1517.
11. McKeith IG, Galasko D, Kosaka K, et al. Consensus guidelines for the clinical and pathologic diagnosis of dementia with Lewy bodies (DLB): Report of the Consortium on DLB International Workshop. *Neurology* 1996;47:1113–1124.
12. Louis E, Klatka LA, Liu Y, et al. Comparison of extrapyramidal features in 31 pathologically confirmed cases of diffuse Lewy body disease and 34 pathologically confirmed cases of Parkinson's disease. *Neurology* 1997;48:376–380.
13. Colcher A, Simuni LZ. Other Parkinson syndromes. *Neurol Clin* 2001;19:629–649.
14. McKeith IG, Del Ser T, Spano P, et al. Efficacy of rivastigmine in dementia with Lewy bodies: a randomised, double-blind, placebo-controlled international study. *Lancet* 2000;356:2031–2036.
15. Miyasaki JM, Martin W, Suchowersky O, et al. Practice parameter: initiation of treatment for Parkinson's disease: an evidence-based review. *Neurology* 2002;58:11–17.
16. Rascol O, Brooks DF, Korczyn AD, et al. A five-year study of the incidence of dyskinesia in patient's with early Parkinson's disease who were treated with ropinirole or levodopa. *N Engl J Med* 2000;342:1484–1491.

Appendixes

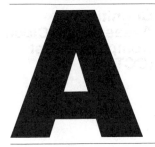

Cognitive Assessment: Modified Short Blessed Test (mSBT)

Patient's Name: _____ DOB: _____ Date: _____

COGNITIVE SCREEN (Short Blessed)	Max error	Error score	× weight =	Sub-score
1. What year is it now?_____	1	_____	4	_____
2. What month is it now?_____	1	_____	3	_____
Repeat this phrase after me and remember it: John Brown, 24 Market Street, Chicago Number of trials to learning: _____				
3. About what time is it without looking at your watch? (within 1 hour) Response _____ Actual Time _____	1	_____	3	_____
4. Count backward from 20 down to 1. Mark correctly sequenced #s. 20 19 18 17 16 15 14 13 12 11 10 9 8 7 6 5 4 3 2 1	2	____(a)	2	_____
5. Say the months of the year in reverse. D N O S A JL JU MY AP M F J Time _____ (Sec.)	2	____(a)	2	_____
6. Repeat the name and address I asked you to remember. John Brown, 24 Market Street, Chicago	5	____(b)	2	_____

TOTAL WEIGHTED ERROR SCORE_____

CENTRAL PROCESSING TIME (#5) _____

(a) Scoring: 0 = no errors, 1 = 1 error, 2 = 2 or more errors.
(b) An answer of either Market or Market Street is acceptable.
_____/ 28 Points – Total Score = A total weighted error score of 9 or greater indicates a need for further assessment.
From Blessed G, Tomlinson BE, Roth M. The association between quantitative measures of dementia and of senile change in the cerebral grey matter of elderly subjects. *Br J Psychiatry* 1968;114:797–811; and Ball LJ, Bisher GB, Birge SJ. A simple test of central processing speed: an extension of the Short Blessed Test. *J Am Geriatr Soc* 1999;47:1359–1363, with permission.

Cognitive Assessment: Clock Completion Test (CCT)

Patient's name: _____ Date of birth: _____ Date: _____

Instructions: Have the patient fill in the numbers on the clock:

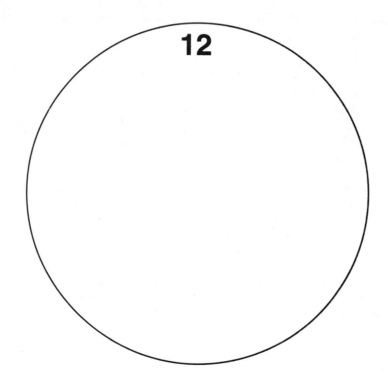

Patient's score: _____ / 7 points

SCORING

The CCT is scored by dividing the predrawn circle, 3.5 in. in diameter, into four equal quadrants oriented through the predrawn "12." Any number on a quadrant line is placed in the clockwise quadrant. The patient is given full credit for each quadrant containing three numbers (see diagram; best possible score of 7 points). A patient has approximately an 80% chance of having Alzheimer's disease if he or she has more or less than three numbers in the fourth clockwise quadrant.

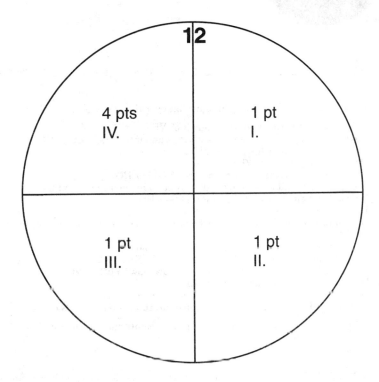

From Watson YI, Arfken CL, Birge SL. Clock completion: an objective screening test for dementia. *J Am Geriatr Soc* 1993;41:1235–1240, with permission.

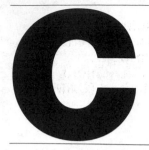

Depression Screen: Geriatric Depression Scale (Short Form)

Patient's name: _____ Date of birth: _____ Date: _____

Choose the best answer for how you have felt over the past week:

1. Are you basically satisfied with your life? YES or **NO**
2. Have you dropped many of your activities and interests? **YES** or NO
3. Do you feel that your life is empty? **YES** or NO
4. Do you often get bored? **YES** or NO
5. Are you in good spirits most of the time? YES or **NO**
6. Are you afraid that something bad is going to happen to you? **YES** or NO
7. Do you feel happy most of the time? YES or **NO**
8. Do you often feel helpless? **YES** or NO
9. Do you prefer staying at home rather than going out and doing new things? **YES** or NO
10. Do you feel you have more problems with memory than most? **YES** or NO
11. Do you think it is wonderful to be alive now? YES or **NO**
12. Do you feel pretty worthless the way you are now? **YES** or NO
13. Do you feel full of energy? YES or **NO**
14. Do you feel that your situation is hopeless? **YES** or NO
15. Do you think that most people are better off than you are? **YES** or NO

Score 1 point for each bold answer. More than 5 points suggests depression.

Patient's score: _____ / 15

From Sheikh JI, Yesavage JA. Geriatric Depression Scale: recent evidence and development of a shorter version. *Clin Gerontol* 1986;5:165–172, with permission.

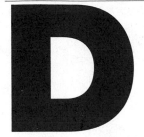

Delirium Assessment: Confusion Assessment Method (CAM)

Patient's name: _____ Date of birth: _____ Date: _____

ACUTE ONSET

1. Is there evidence of an acute change in mental status from the patient's baseline?

    __ yes __ no

INATTENTION

2A. Did the patient have difficulty focusing attention, for example, being easily distractible or having difficulty keeping track of what was said?

    __ not present at any time during interview (go to item 3)
    __ present at some time during interview, but in mild form (go to items 2B and 2C)
    __ present at some time during interview, in marked form (go to items 2B and 2C)
    __ uncertain (go to item 3)

2B. Did this behavior fluctuate during the interview—that is, tend to come and go or increase and decrease in severity?

    __ yes __ no __ uncertain __ N/A

2C. Please describe this behavior.

DISORGANIZED THINKING

3. Was the patient's thinking disorganized or incoherent, such as rambling or irrelevant conversation, unclear or illogical flow of ideas, or unpredictable switching from subject to subject?

    __ yes __ no

ALTERED LEVEL OF CONSCIOUSNESS

4. Overall, how would you rate this patient's level of consciousness?

    __ alert (normal)
    __ vigilant (hyperalert, overly sensitive to environmental stimuli, startled very easily)
    __ lethargic (drowsy, easily aroused)
    __ stupor (difficult to arouse)
    __ coma (unarousable)
    __ uncertain

DISORIENTATION

5. Was the patient disoriented at any time during the interview, such as thinking that he or she was somewhere other than the hospital, using the wrong bed, or misjudging the time of day?

___ yes ___ no

MEMORY IMPAIRMENT

6. Did the patient demonstrate any memory problems during the interview, such as inability to remember events in the hospital or difficulty remembering instructions?

___ yes ___ no

PERCEPTUAL DISTURBANCES

7. Did the patient have any evidence of perceptual disturbances, for example, hallucinations, illusions, or misinterpretations (such as thinking something was moving when it was not)?

___ yes ___ no

PSYCHOMOTOR AGITATION

8. Part 1. At any time during the interview, did the patient have an unusually increased level of motor activity, such as restlessness, picking at bedclothes, tapping fingers, or making frequent sudden changes in position?

___ yes ___ no

9. Part 2. At any time during the interview, did the patient have an unusually decreased level of motor activity, such as sluggishness, staring into space, staying in one position for a long time, or moving very slowly?

___ yes ___ no

ALTERED SLEEP-WAKE CYCLE

10. Did the patient have evidence of disturbance of the sleep-wake cycle, such as excessive daytime sleepiness with insomnia at night?

___ yes ___ no

SCORING

To have a positive CAM result, the patient must demonstrate:

1. Presence of acute onset and fluctuating course ___ yes ___ no

   and

2. Inattention ___ yes ___ no

   and either

3. Disorganized thinking ___ yes ___ no

   or

4. Altered level of consciousness ___ yes ___ no

Patient's CAM result: ___ Positive ___ Negative

Courtesy of S. Inouye, M.D., M.P.H., Yale University School of Medicine, New Haven, CT.

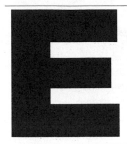

Polypharmacy: Common Formulas and Cytochrome P450 Drug Interactions

FORMULAS

Volume of distribution = ratio of the mass of the drug in the body/concentration in the blood

T $\frac{1}{2}$ = 0.693 × Vd / plasma clearance

CrCl =

$$\frac{(140-\text{age}) \times \text{lean body weight (LBW) (kg) (multiply by 0.85 for women if using actual weight)}}{72 \times \text{serum Cr}}$$

Normal CrCl range in men: 100–125 mL/min
Normal CrCl range in women: 85–100 mL/min

LBW = IBW (ideal body weight) + 0.4 (actual body weight – IBW)

Male IBW = 50 kg + (2.3 kg) × (each in. of height >5 ft)

Female IBW = 45.5 kg + (2.3 kg) × (each in. of height >5 ft)

CYTOCHROME P1A2 DRUG INTERACTIONS

Substrates	Inhibitors	Inducers
Theophylline	Fluvoxamine	Smoking
R-Warfarin	Ciprofloxacin	Phenobarbital
Tricyclic antidepressants	Cimetidine	Phenytoin
Diazepam	Macrolides	Rifampin
Haloperidol	Grapefruit juice	
	Isoniazid	
	Ketoconazole	

CYTOCHROME P2C9/2C19 DRUG INTERACTIONS

Substrates	Inhibitors	Inducers
S-Warfarin	Amiodarone	Carbamazepine
Phenytoin	Fluvoxamine	Phenytoin
Diazepam	Fluoxetine	Phenobarbital
Omeprazole	Sertraline	Rifampin
Tricyclic antidepressants	Cimetidine	
	Omeprazole	
	Chloramphenicol	
	Zafirlukast	
	Fluconazole	
	Isoniazid	

CYTOCHROME P2D6 DRUG INTERACTIONS

Substrates	Inhibitors	Inducers
Opiates	Quinidine	Rifampin
Antiarrhythmics	SSRIs	Carbamazepine
Tricyclic antidepressants	Cimetidine	Phenobarbital
Antipsychotics	Amiodarone	Phenytoin
Beta blockers		Primidone

CYTOCHROME P3A4 DRUG INTERACTIONS

Substrates	Inhibitors	Inducers
Cisapride	Macrolides	Rifampin
Alprazolam	Azole antifungals	Carbamazepine
Midazolam	SSRIs	Phenobarbital
Statins	Nefazodone	Phenytoin
Calcium-channel blockers	Amiodarone	Primidone
R-Warfarin	Metronidazole	Dexamethasone
Prednisone	Grapefruit juice	
Dexamethasone		
Estrogens		
Carbamazepine		
Quinidine		
Lidocaine		
Disopyramide		

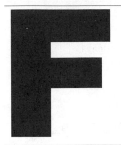

Weight Loss and Nutrition Tools: Appetite and Nutrition Assessment

APPETITE ASSESSMENT

Patient's name: _____ Date of birth: _____ Date: _____ Weight: _____

	1	2	3	4	5
My appetite is...	Very poor	Poor	Average	Good	Very good
When I eat, I feel full after...	Eating only a few mouthfuls	Eating approximately one-third of a plate full	Eating more than one-half a plate full	Eating most of the food	Hardly ever
I feel hungry...	Never	Occasionally	Some of the time	Most of the time	All of the time
Food tastes...	Very poor	Poor	Average	Good	Very good
Compared to when I was 50 yrs old, food tastes...	Much worse	Worse	Just as good	Better	Much better
Normally, I eat...	Less than one full meal a day	One meal a day	Two meals a day	Three meals a day	More than three meals a day, including snacks
I feel sick or nauseated when I eat...	Most times	Often	Sometimes	Rarely	Never
Most of the time my mood is...	Very sad	Sad	Neither sad nor happy	Happy	Very happy

Total Score: _____ / 40
From Thomas DR, Morley JE. Regulation of appetite in older adults. The Council for Nutritional:Clinical Strategies in Long-Term Care. Supplement to *Annals of Long Term Care*, with permission.

BRIEF NUTRITION ASSESSMENT

	At age 50	Reported current	Actual current
Weight	_____	_____	_____
Height	_____	_____	_____

Loss of 10 or more lbs in last 6 mos: Yes ___ No ___

Dentition: adequate for chewing: Yes __ No __, Denture: Yes __ No __, Fit: Yes __ No __

Albumin: _____ Calcium: _____ Phosphorus: _____ Cholesterol: _____

Absolute lymphocyte count: _____ Hgb: _____ Mean cell volume: _____

25-hydroxyvitamin D: _____

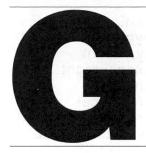

Androgen Deficiency in Aging Men (ADAM) Questionnaire

Patient's name: _____ Date of birth: _____ Date: _____

	Yes	No
1. Do you have a decrease in libido (sex drive)?		
2. Do you have a lack of energy?		
3. Do you have a decrease in strength or endurance?		
4. Have you lost height?		
5. Have you noticed a decreased enjoyment of life?		
6. Are you sad or grumpy?		
7. Are your erections less strong?		
8. Are you falling asleep after dinner?		
9. Have you noted a recent deterioration in your ability to play sports?		
10. Has there been a recent deterioration in your work performance?		

INTERPRETATION

Positive responses to items 1, 7, or a combination of any three or more is suggestive of androgen deficiency.

From Morley JE, Charlton E, Patrick P, et al. Validation of a screening questionnaire for androgen deficiency in aging males. *Metabolism* 2000;49(9):1239–1242, with permission.

Total testosterone: _____ Date: _____

Free or bioavailable testosterone: _____ Date: _____

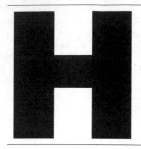

Benign Prostatic Hyperplasia (BPH) Symptom Assessment: American Urological Association (AUA) Symptom Score

Patient's name: _____ Date of birth: _____ Date: _____

Question	Not at all	Less than one time in five	Less than one-half the time	Approximately one-half the time	More than one-half the time	Almost always
Over the past month, how often have you had a sensation of not emptying your bladder completely after you finished urinating?	0	1	2	3	4	5
Over the past month, how often have you had to urinate again <2 hrs after you finished urinating?	0	1	2	3	4	5
Over the past month, how often have you stopped and started again several times when you urinated?	0	1	2	3	4	5
Over the past month, how often have you found it difficult to postpone urination?	0	1	2	3	4	5
Over the past month, how often have you had a weak urine stream?	0	1	2	3	4	5

(*continued*)

Question	Not at all	Less than one time in five	Less than one-half the time	Approximately one-half the time	More than one-half the time	Almost always
Over the past month, how often have you had to push or strain to begin urination?	0	1	2	3	4	5
Over the past month, how many times most typically did you get up to urinate from the time you went to bed at night until the time you got up in the morning?	0	1	2	3	4	5

Patient's score: _____ / 35
Current medications for BPH: _____

SCORING

A score of 0–7 equates with mild symptoms, 8–19 with moderate symptoms, and > 19 with severe symptoms.

From Barry MJ, et al. The American Urological Association symptom index for benign prostatic hyperplasia. *J Urol* 1992;148:1549–1557, with permission.

Erectile Dysfunction Symptom Assessment: Sexual Health Inventory for Men (SHIM)

Patient's name: _____ Date of birth: _____ Date: _____

	Over the past 6 mos:					
1.	How do you rate your **confidence** that you could get and keep an erection?	Very low 1	Low 2	Moderate 3	High 4	Very high 5
2.	When you had erections with sexual stimulation, how often were your erections hard enough for penetration?	Almost never/ never 1	A few times (much less than half the time) 2	Sometimes (about half the time) 3	Most times (much more than half the time) 4	Almost always/ always 5
3.	During sexual intercourse, **how often** were you able to maintain your erection after you had penetrated (entered) your partner?	Almost never/ never 1	A few times (much less than half the time) 2	Sometimes (about half the time) 3	Most times (much more than half the time) 4	Almost always/ always 5
4.	During sexual intercourse, how difficult was it to maintain your erection to completion of intercourse?	Extremely difficult 1	Very difficult 2	Difficult 3	Slightly difficult 4	Not difficult 5
5.	When you attempted sexual intercourse, how often was it satisfactory for you?	Almost never/ never 1	A few times (much less than half the time) 2	Sometimes (about half the time) 3	Most times (much more than half the time) 4	Almost always/ always 5

Patient's score: _____ / 25

The Sexual Health Inventory for Men (SHIM) is a subset of questions from the IIEF (International Index of Erectile Dysfunction) questionnaire. The IIEF-5 (SHIM) score is the sum of the ordinal responses to the five items: the score can range from 5–25. A score of <22 may indicate a problem.

SHIM GRADE OF ERECTILE DYSFUNCTION (ED) SEVERITY

SHIM score	ED severity
22–25	None
17–21	Mild ED
12–16	Mild–moderate ED
8–11	Moderate ED
1–7	Severe ED

From Rosen RC, et al. Development and evaluation of an abridged, 5-item version of the International Index of Erectile Function (IIEF-5) as a diagnostic tool for erectile dysfunction. *Int J Impot Res* 1999;11:319–326, with permission.

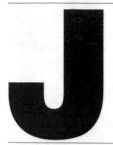

Visual Acuity Assessment: Rosenbaum Vision Screen

ROSENBAUM POCKET VISION SCREENER

			distance equivalent
95			20/800

		Point	Jaeger	
874				20/400
2843		26	16	20/200
638 E Ш Ξ X O O		14	10	20/100
8 7 4 5 Ξ ᛖ Ш O X O		10	7	20/70
6 3 9 2 5 ᛖ E Ξ X O X		8	5	20/50
4 2 8 3 6 5 Ш E ᛖ O X O		6	3	20/40
3 7 4 2 5 8 ᛝ Ш ᛝ X X O		5	2	20/30
9 3 7 8 2 6 Ш ᛖ E X O O		4	1	20/25
4 2 8 7 3 9 E Ш ᛖ O O X		3	1+	20/20

Card is held in good light 14 inches from eye. Record vision for each eye separately with and without glasses. Presbyopic patients should read thru bifocal segment. Check myopes with glasses only.

DESIGN COURTESY J. G. ROSENBAUM, M.D

PUPIL GAUGE (mm.)

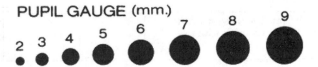

2   3   4   5   6   7   8   9

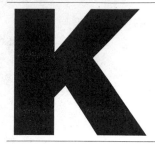

Hearing Loss Screening: Hearing Handicap Inventory in the Elderly—Screen and Whisper Test

Patient's name: _____ Date of birth: _____ Date: _____

HEARING HANDICAP INVENTORY IN THE ELDERLY—SCREEN

	Yes (4 points)	Sometimes (2 points)	No (1 point)
Does a hearing problem cause you to feel embarrassed when meeting new people?			
Does a hearing problem cause you to feel frustrated when talking to members of your family?			
Do you have difficulty hearing when someone speaks in a whisper?			
Do you feel handicapped by a hearing problem?			
Does a hearing problem cause you difficulty when visiting friends, relatives, or neighbors?			
Does a hearing problem cause you to attend religious services less often than you would like?			
Does a hearing problem cause you to have arguments with family members?			
Does a hearing problem cause you difficulty when you are listening to the TV or radio?			
Do you feel that any difficulty with your hearing limits or hampers your personal or social life?			
Does a hearing problem cause you difficulty when in a restaurant with relatives or friends?			

Patient's score: _____ / 40

Scoring: 0–8, no self perceived handicap; 10–22, mild to moderate handicap; 24–40, significant handicap.
From Ventry IM, Weinstein BE. Identification of elderly people with hearing problems. *ASHA* 1983;25(7):37–42, with permission.

WHISPER TEST

With the subject sitting, ask the subject to place a finger in his or her left ear canal and move it up and down repeatedly. At a distance of 2 ft on the side of the right ear, softly whisper a three-syllable word and ask him or her to repeat it (i.e., 99). Repeat a different three-syllable word if he or she could not repeat what you said (i.e., 37). Document if the subject could repeat at least one of the whispered words. Repeat the procedure with the left ear while the subject occludes the right ear.

RIGHT EAR: NORMAL/ABNORMAL   LEFT EAR: NORMAL/ABNORMAL

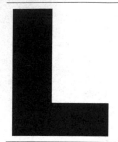

Pressure Ulcer Risk Assessment: Braden Risk Assessment Scale

Patient's name: _____		Date of birth: _____		Date: _____		Score
Sensory perception: Ability to respond meaningfully to pressure-related discomfort.	**1. Completely limited:** Unresponsive (does not moan, flinch, or grasp) to painful stimuli owing to diminished level of consciousness or sedation OR limited ability to feel pain over most of body surface.	**2. Very limited:** Responds only to painful stimuli. Cannot communicate discomfort except by moaning or restlessness OR has a sensory impairment that limits the ability to feel pain or discomfort over one-half of body.	**3. Slightly limited:** Responds to verbal commands but cannot always communicate discomfort or need to be turned OR has some sensory impairment that limits ability to feel pain or discomfort in 1 or 2 extremities.	**4. No impairment:** Responds to verbal commands, has no sensory deficit that would limit ability to feel or voice pain or discomfort.		
Moisture: Degree to which skin is exposed to moisture.	**1. Constantly moist:** Skin is kept moist almost constantly by perspiration, urine, etc. Dampness is detected every time patient is moved or turned.	**2. Moist:** Skin is often but not always moist. Linen must be changed at least once a shift.	**3. Occasionally moist:** Skin is occasionally moist, requiring an extra linen change at least once a day.	**4. Rarely moist:** Skin is usually dry; linen requires changing only at routine intervals.		
Activity: Degree of physical activity.	**1. Bedfast:** Confined to bed.	**2. Chairfast:** Ability to walk severely limited or nonexistent. Cannot bear weight and/or must be assisted into chair or wheelchair.	**3. Walks occasionally:** Walks occasionally during day but for very short distances, with or without assistance. Spends majority of each shift in bed or chair.	**4. Walks frequently:** Walks outside the room at least twice a day and inside room at least once every 2 hrs during waking hours.		
Mobility: Ability to change and control body position.	**1. Completely immobile:** Does not make even slight changes in body or extremity position without assistance.	**2. Very limited:** Makes occasional slight changes in body or extremity position but unable to make frequent or significant changes independently.	**3. Slightly limited:** Makes frequent although slight changes in body or extremity position independently.	**4. No limitations:** Makes major and frequent changes in position without assistance.		

	1. Very poor	2. Probably inadequate	3. Adequate	4. Excellent	Score
Nutrition: Usual food intake pattern.	**1. Very poor:** Never eats a complete meal. Rarely eats more than one-third of any food offered. Eats ≤ 2 servings of protein (meat or dairy products) per day. Takes liquids poorly. Does not take a liquid dietary supplement OR is NPO and/or maintained on clear liquids or IV for >5 days.	**2. Probably inadequate:** Rarely eats a complete meal and generally eats only approximately one-half of any food offered. Protein intake includes only 3 servings of meat or dairy products per day. Occasionally will take a dietary supplement OR receives less-than-optimum amount of liquid diet or tube feeding.	**3. Adequate:** Eats more than one-half of most meals. Eats a total of 4 servings of protein (meat or dairy products) each day. Occasionally will refuse a meal but will usually take a supplement if offered OR is on a tube feeding or TPN regimen, which probably meets most of nutritional needs.	**4. Excellent:** Eats most of every meal. Never refuses a meal. Usually eats a total of 4 or more servings of meat and dairy products. Occasionally eats between meals. Does not require supplementation.	
Friction and shear	**1. Problem:** Requires moderate to maximum assistance in moving. Complete lifting without sliding against sheets is impossible. Frequently slides down in bed or chair, requiring frequent repositioning with maximum assistance. Spasticity, contractures, or agitation leads to almost constant friction.	**2. Potential problem:** Moves feebly or requires minimum assistance. During a move, skin probably slides to some extent against sheets, chair, restraints, or other devices. Maintains relatively good position in chair or bed most of the time but occasionally slides down.	**3. No apparent problem:** Moves in bed and in chair independently and has sufficient muscle strength to lift up completely during move. Maintains good position in bed or chair at all times.		
				Total Score	

Patient's score: ____ / 23
Scoring: ≤ 10, high risk; 11–16, moderate risk; ≥ 17, low risk.
Interventions taken (check appropriate actions for all patients with score of ≤ 16):
Air mattress: _____ Waffle boots: _____ Dietitian: _____ Wound nurse: _____
Weekly weights: _____ Air seat cushion: _____ Physical therapy: _____
Courtesy of Barbara Braden and Nancy Bergstrom. Copyright, 1988.

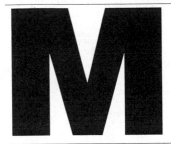

Functional Assessment: Katz Index of Activities of Daily Living (ADLs)

Patient's name: _____ Date of birth: _____ Date: _____

Source: _____ Score: _____

INSTRUCTIONS

Indicate the levels of assistance needed with the following six ADLs by circling the score that most closely describes the patient.

	Score
Bathing (either sponge bath, tub bath, or shower)	
Receives no assistance (gets in and out of tub by self is usual means of bathing).	3
Receives assistance in bathing only one part of body, such as the back or a leg.	2
Receives assistance in bathing more than one part of body or is not bathed.	1
Continence	
Controls urination and bowel movement completely by self.	3
Has occasional "accidents."	2
Needs supervision to keep urine or bowel control, uses catheter, or is incontinent.	1
Dressing (gets clothes from closets and drawers, including underclothes, outer garments; uses fasteners, including braces, if worn)	
Gets clothes and gets completely dressed without assistance.	3
Gets clothes and gets dressed without assistance except in tying shoes.	2
Receives assistance in getting clothes or getting dressed or stays partly or completely undressed.	1
Feeding	
Feeds self without assistance.	3
Feeds self except for assistance in cutting meat or buttering bread.	2
Receives assistance in feeding or is fed partly or completely by NG or gastric tubes or IV fluids.	1
Toileting	
Goes to "toilet room," cleans self, and arranges clothes without assistance (may use objects for support, such as cane, walker, or wheelchair and may manage night bedpan or commode and empty same in morning).	3

	Score
Receives assistance in going to "toilet room," cleaning self, or arranging clothes after elimination or receives assistance in using night bedpan or commode.	2
Does not go to room termed "toilet" for the elimination process.	1

Transferring

Moves in and out of bed or chair without assistance (may use object for support such as cane or walker).	3
Moves in and out of bed or chair with assistance.	2
Does not get out of bed.	1

Total score

Adapted from Katz S, Ford AB, Moskowitz RW, et al. Studies of illness in the aged. The index of ADL: a standardized measure of biological and psychosocial function. *JAMA* 1963;185:914–919.

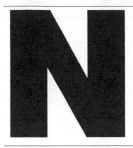

Functional Assessment: Lawton Index of Instrumental Activities of Daily Living (IADLs)

Patient's name: _____ Date of birth: _____ Date: _____

Source: _____ Score: _____

INSTRUCTIONS

Indicate the levels of assistance needed with the following eight IADLs by circling the score that most closely describes the patient.

	Score
Uses the telephone	
Without help	3
With some help	2
Completely unable to use the telephone	1
Gets to places out of walking distance	
Without help	3
With some help	2
Completely unable to travel unless special arrangements are made	1
Goes shopping for groceries	
Without help	3
With some help	2
Completely unable to do any shopping	1
Prepares own meals	
Without help	3
With some help	2
Completely unable to prepare any meals	1
Does own housework	
Without help	3
With some help	2
Completely unable to do housework	1
Does own handyman work	
Without help	3
With some help	2
Completely unable to do handyman work	1

	Score
Does own laundry	
Without help	3
With some help	2
Completely unable to do laundry	1
Takes own medication	
Without help (in the right dose at the right time)	3
With some help (takes medicine if someone prepares it or reminds them)	2
Completely unable to take own medication	1
Manages own money	
Without help	3
With some help	2
Completely unable to handle money	1
Total score	

Adapted from Lawton MP. Assessment of older people: self-maintaining and instrumental activities of daily living. *Gerontologist* 1969;9:179–185.

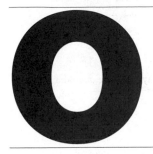

Parkinson's Disease Motor Scale: Unified Parkinson's Disease Rating Scale (UPDRS), Subscale III

SPEECH

0: Normal
1: Slight loss of expression, diction, volume
2: Monotone, slurred but understandable, moderately impaired
3: Marked impairment, difficult to understand
4: Unintelligible

FACIAL EXPRESSION

0: Normal
1: Slight hypomimia, could be poker face
2: Slight but definite abnormal diminution in expression
3: Moderate hypomimia, lips parted some of time
4: Masked or fixed face, lips parted 1/4 in. or more with complete loss of expression

TREMOR AT REST

Rate face, right upper extremity (RUE), left upper extremity (LUE), right lower extremity (RLE), left lower extremity (LLE) independently.

0: Absent
1: Slight and infrequent
2: Mild and present most of time
3: Moderate and present most of time
4: Marked and present most of time

ACTION OR POSTURAL TREMOR

Rate RUE and LUE independently.

0: Absent
1: Slight, present with action
2: Moderate, present with action
3: Moderate present with action and posture holding
4: Marked, interferes with feeding

RIGIDITY

Rate neck, RUE, LUE, RLE, and LLE independently.

0: Absent
1: Slight or only with activation of contralateral side
2: Mild/moderate
3: Marked, full range of motion difficult
4: Severe

FINGER TAPS

Rate RUE and LUE independently.

0: Normal
1: Mild slowing, and/or reduction in amp
2: Moderately impaired—definite and early fatiguing, may have occasional arrests
3: Severely impaired—frequent hesitations and arrests
4: Can barely perform the task

HAND MOVEMENTS

Open and close hands in rapid succession. Rate RUE and LUE independently.

0: Normal
1: Mild slowing and/or reduction in amp
2: Moderately impaired—definite and early fatiguing, may have occasional arrests
3: Severely impaired—frequent hesitations and arrests
4: Can barely perform the task

RAPID ALTERNATING MOVEMENTS (PRONATE AND SUPINATE HANDS)

Rate RUE and LUE independently.

0: Normal
1: Mild slowing and/or reduction in amp
2: Moderately impaired—definite and early fatiguing, may have occasional arrests
3: Severely impaired—frequent hesitations and arrests
4: Can barely perform the task

LEG AGILITY

Tap heel on ground; amplitude should be 3 in. Rate RLE and LLE independently.

0: Normal
1: Mild slowing and/or reduction in amp
2: Moderately impaired—definite and early fatiguing, may have occasional arrests
3: Severely impaired—frequent hesitations and arrests
4: Can barely perform the task

ARISING FROM CHAIR

Patient arises with arms folded across chest.

0: Normal
1: Slow, may need more than one attempt
2: Pushes self up from arms or seat
3: Tends to fall back, may need multiple tries but can arise without assistance
4: Unable to arise without help

POSTURE

0: Normal erect
1: Slightly stooped, could be normal for older person
2: Definitely abnormal, moderately stooped, may lean to one side
3: Severely stooped with kyphosis
4: Marked flexion with extreme abnormality of posture

GAIT

0: Normal
1: Walks slowly, may shuffle with short steps, no festination or propulsion
2: Walks with difficulty, little or no assistance, some festination, short steps or propulsion
3: Severe disturbance, frequent assistance
4: Cannot walk

POSTURAL STABILITY (PULL TEST OR RETROPULSION TEST)

0: Normal
1: Recovers unaided
2: Would fall if not caught
3: Falls spontaneously
4: Unable to stand

BODY BRADYKINESIA/HYPOKINESIA

0: None
1: Minimal slowness, could be normal, deliberate character
2: Mild slowness and poverty of movement, definitely abnormal, or decelerated amplitude of movement
3: Moderate slowness, poverty, or small amplitude
4: Marked slowness, poverty, or amplitude

From Fahn S, Marsden CD, Calne DB, et al., eds. *Recent developments in Parkinson's disease*, Vol. 2. Florham Park, NJ: Macmillan Health Care Information, 1987:153–163, 293–304, with permission.

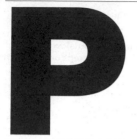

Selected Topics and Useful Resources for Older Adults

Tammy L. Lin

ADVANCE PLANNING

A **health care advance directive** is a document that a patient can leave instructions about the type of health care desired if he or she is not able to make or communicate about decisions in the future. He or she is able to give health care decision-making powers to an "agent" or "proxy." There are two main types of advance directives. A **Living Will** typically states a patient's wishes about life-sustaining medical treatments if he or she is terminally ill. A **Health Care Power of Attorney** typically allows a patient to name someone else to make health care decisions if he or she is unable to do so. It is not limited to patients with terminal illnesses. These documents allow patients to keep control over critical health care decisions and may relieve family members and loved ones of the stresses of making these types of decisions. Health Care Advance Directives are valid in every state, and a patient has the right to change or invalidate it at any time. Physicians should speak with their patients earlier rather than later about the types of medical problems they may face based on their current health status and encourage creation of a health care advance directive. Discussion about **code status** is also vital. The American Medical Association (AMA) has created a booklet entitled *Shape Your Health Care Future with HEALTH CARE ADVANCE DIRECTIVES* (http://www.ama-assn.org/public/booklets/livgwill.htm), which may be helpful for patients and physicians and contains sample documents. In addition to local agencies on aging, bar associations, medical societies, or hospital associations, more state-by-state information or information about creating a health care advance directive can be obtained by contacting the following:

Legal Counsel for the Elderly (LCE)
American Association of Retired Persons (AARP)
P.O. Box 96474
Washington, DC 20090-6474
Phone: (202) 434-2120
(http://www.aarp.org/lce/)

Choice in Dying, Inc.
200 Varick Street
New York, NY 10014-4810
Phone: 1-800-989-WILL
(http://www.partnershipforcaring.org/)

HOSPICE CARE

Hospice care can provide coordinated support services for those who are terminally ill and their families. The goal in hospice care is to provide an improved quality of life in patients with limited life expectancy (usually ≤ 6 mos) and a comfortable death. Nurses skilled in pain and symptom management, home health aides, social workers, volunteers, chaplains, and the patient's physician often form the interdisciplinary team delivering care in the home, nursing home, or hospital. Medicare covers hospice benefits in qualified patients. More information can be obtained from the National Hospice and Palliative Care Organization (http://www.nhpco.org/).

MEDICARE AND MEDICAID

Medicare and Medicaid benefits are available for qualified patients (people >65 yrs old, some people with disabilities, people 65 yrs old, people with end-stage renal disease). Please see Chap. 2, Settings for Geriatric Care, for more details. Those who have paid Medicare taxes while they were working automatically qualify for Part A (Hospital Insurance) when they turn 65 yrs old. A patient may still be able to buy Part A even if he or she (or spouse) did not pay Medicare taxes previously. The local Social Security office or the Social Security Administration (phone: 1-800-772-1213) can be contacted for more information about buying Part A. In addition, more general information and publications can be obtained by visiting the Medical Consumer Information Web site at http://www.medicare.gov/, which can be read in English, Spanish, and Chinese, or by calling 1-800-MEDICARE. Information about prescription drug assistance for those with low income or specific diseases can be found in the above site (http://www.medicare.gov/AssistancePrograms/TabTop). Information about Medicaid can be found at http://cms.hhs.gov/.

SAFETY AND HOME HEALTH CARE

Injury prevention is a significant concern in the older adult population. Any medical risk factors for falls should be addressed and treated appropriately. Side effects from medications, visual impairment, or specific diseases (e.g., osteoporosis, cerebrovascular accidents, gait or balance disorders) often contribute to fall risk. Mobility screening and an environmental assessment can also be performed. A **home safety assessment** can be performed by occupational therapists skilled in evaluating extrinsic risk factors in the home. There are also occupational therapists who specialize in evaluating older drivers for safety on the road and appropriate assistive devices. Physical therapists are skilled in strength, gait, and balance training; evaluation of assistive devices; and rehabilitation efforts.

Many services can be delivered in the home environment. The Visiting Nurse Associations of America (http://www.vnaa.org/) help to provide such services. Their mission is to support community-based visiting nurses in providing **home health care and hospice care** through skilled nursing; therapy services (physical therapy, occupational therapy, speech therapy), and home health aide/personal care to elderly, children, homebound, disabled, and terminally ill patients. Home health care services required after a hospital stay (e.g., home infusions, assistance with medications, physical therapy) can often be arranged through a social worker or case coordinator before discharge.

There may also be situations in which a patient's safety is at risk, and physicians have reporting requirements. The duty to report **unsafe older drivers** varies between states and local areas. Some states have mandatory reporting requirements. Specific information can be found through the National Highway Traffic Safety Administration (NHTSA) Web site (http://www.nhtsa.dot.gov/). More educational information on this topic can be found in the older driver safety resources from the AMA (http://www.ama-assn.org/ama/pub/category/8925.html) and NHTSA (http://www.nhtsa.dot.gov/people/injury/olddrive/). In addition, the AARP sponsors a program called AARP 55-ALIVE (http://www.aarp.org/drive/) to help older adults improve driving skills.

In cases of **elder abuse** in the home or in institutions, physicians have a responsibility to report the circumstances to Adult Protective Services (APS). Each state has a toll-free hotline to report abuse or neglect, and these numbers can be obtained through the National Center on Elder Abuse (http://www.elderabusecenter.org/). Inquire about any abuse or neglect (physical, psychological, or financial) regularly, and document any findings carefully.

SLEEP DISORDERS

Sleep disorders can be very disruptive in the older adult population. Types of problems may include insomnia, frequent or early awakening, excessive sleep, or abnormal behaviors associated with sleep. The causes for these disorders may be medical, psychological, or functional, and a tailored history, physical exam, and workup often uncover them. Some patients may need to be referred for further studies. Common reasons for disordered sleep include symptoms from chronic illnesses, chronic pain, sleep apnea, restless less syndrome, stimulants, substance abuse, sedentary lifestyle, depression, frequent urination, poor sleep hygiene, and dementia. Counseling on proper sleep hygiene, relaxation, and treatment of underlying medical conditions can usually promote more satisfying sleep. Long-term insomnia treatment with medications (e.g., benzodiazepines or sedating antihistamines) is not recommended and may be harmful. Antidepressants that are non-habit forming, such as amitriptyline (10–25 mg PO qhs) or trazodone (50 mg PO qhs), may be helpful in the short term. Similarly, zolpidem (Ambien) (2.5–10 mg PO qhs) may be another short-term alternative. Additional information for physicians and patients can be found at the following Web sites: the American Sleep Disorders Association (http://www.asda.org), Medline plus (http://www.nlm.nih.gov/medlineplus/ency/article/000064.htm), the National Sleep Foundation (http://www.sleepfoundation.org/), and Sleep Home Pages (http://www.sleephomepages.org/).

SUBSTANCE ABUSE

Substance abuse is often not recognized in older adults and can have severe consequences in terms of health, quality-of-life, and medical costs. Substance abuse can stem from chronic or recurrent patterns, use of medications required for chronic medical conditions, loss of loved ones, or lifestyle changes after age 65 yrs. Chronic pain, depression, polypharmacy, and age-related changes in drug metabolism are also risk factors. The most common substances abused include alcohol, tobacco, and prescription drugs (especially benzodiazepines). A careful history and appropriate screening (with family members or friends if appropriate) during visits can often uncover a substance abuse problem. Patients may also present with symptoms such as sleep disturbance, hypertension, depressed mood, anxiety, or problems with sexual function. Effective treatments are available, and there are many resources and rehabilitation programs to choose from depending on the type of problem. One place to start is the U.S. Department of Health and Human Services and Substance Abuse and Mental Health Services Administration's (SAMHSA) National Clearinghouse for Alcohol and Drug Information Substance Abuse Resource Guide: Older Americans. It contains information on publications and has links to organizations and resources. The guide can be found at (http://www.health.org/govpubs/ms443/) or by calling 1-800-729-6686. Another place to find similar information is the SAMHSA Web site at http://www.samhsa.gov.

OTHER RESOURCES AND WEB SITES FOR PATIENTS AND PROVIDERS
General Resources

Administration on Aging (http://www.aoa.dhhs.gov/) or 1-202-619-0724
American Association of Retired Persons (http://www.aarp.org/) or 1-800-993-7222
American Geriatric Society (http://www.americangeriatrics.org/)
Area Agency on Aging (http://www.n4a.org/) or 1-800-677-1116
Meals on Wheels Association of America (http://www.mowaa.org/index.shtml) or 1-703-548-5558 National Association of Social Workers (http://www.naswdc.org/)
National Institute on Aging (http://www.nih.gov/nia) or 1-301-496-1752

Resources for Selected Diseases

American Cancer Society (http://www.cancer.org)
American Heart Association (http://www.americanheart.org)
American Stroke Association (http://www.strokeassociation.org)
Alzheimer's Disease and Education and Referral Center (http://www.alzheimers.org/)
Family Caregiver Alliance (http://www.caregiver.org/)
National Emphysema Foundation (http://www.emphysemafoundation.org)
National Foundation for Depressive Illness (http://www.depression.org/)

National Institutes of Health Osteoporosis and Related Bone Disease—National Resource Center (http://www.osteo.org/)
Parkinson's Disease Foundation (http://www.pdf.org/)

REFERENCES AND SUGGESTED READINGS

Angelo S. Sleep disorders in the elderly. Medline plus Health Information Web site. Available at: http://www.nlm.nih.gov/medlineplus/ency/article/000064.htm. Accessed October 2003.

Carr D. Geriatrics. In: *The Washington manual of ambulatory therapeutics*. Philadelphia: Lippincott Williams & Wilkins, 2002:653–656.

Center for Medicare and Medicaid Services Web site. Available at: http://www.cms.gov/. Accessed October 2003.

Golladay G, Lin T. Internet medicine and useful websites. In: *The Washington manual of ambulatory therapeutics*. Philadelphia: Lippincott Williams & Wilkins, 2002:680–683.

Medicare Consumer Information Web site. Available at: http://www.medicare.gov/. Accessed October 2003.

National Center on Elder Abuse Web site. Available at: http://www.elderabusecenter.org/. Accessed October 2003.

National Highway Traffic Safety Administration Web site. Available at: http://www.nhtsa. dot.gov/. Accessed October 2003.

Schultz M. Oncology and palliative care. In: *The Washington manual of ambulatory therapeutics*. Philadelphia: Lippincott Williams & Wilkins, 2002:358.

U.S. Department of Health and Human Services and Substance Abuse and Mental Health Services Administration's (SAMHSA) National Clearinghouse for Alcohol and Drug Information Substance Abuse Resource Guide: Older Americans Web site. Available at: http://www.health.org/govpubs/ms443/. Accessed October 2003.

Index

Page numbers followed by *t* indicate tables; numbers followed by *f* indicate figures.